THE CARER'S
COSMETIC
HANDBOOK

of related interest

How to Make Your Care Home Fun
Simple Activities for People of All Abilities
Kenneth Agar
ISBN 978 1 84310 952 5

The Activity Year Book
A Week by Week Guide for Use in Elderly Day and Residential Care
Anni Bowden and Nancy Lewthwaite
ISBN 978 1 84310 963 1

Involving Families in Care Homes
A Relationship-Centred Approach to Dementia Care
Bob Woods, John Keady and Diane Seddon
ISBN 978 1 84310 229 8
Bradford Dementia Group Good Practice Guides

The Pool Activity Level (PAL) Instrument for Occupational Profiling
A Practical Resource for Carers of People with Cognitive Impairment
3rd edition
Jackie Pool
ISBN 978 1 84310 594 7

Understanding Care Homes
A Research and Development Perspective
Edited by Katherine Froggatt, Sue Davies and Julienne Meyer
ISBN 978 1 84310 553 4

Design for Nature in Dementia Care
Garuth Chalfont
ISBN 978 1 84310 571 8
Bradford Dementia Group Good Practice Guides

THE CARER'S COSMETIC HANDBOOK

Simple Health and Beauty Tips for Older Persons

Sharon Tay

Jessica Kingsley Publishers
London and Philadelphia

First published in 2009
by Jessica Kingsley Publishers
116 Pentonville Road
London N1 9JB, UK
and
400 Market Street, Suite 400
Philadelphia, PA 19106, USA

www.jkp.com

Library of Congress Cataloging in Publication Data

Tay, Sharon.
    The carer's cosmetic handbook : simple health and beauty tips for older persons / Sharon
Tay.
        p. cm.
    Includes bibliographical references.
    ISBN 978-1-84310-973-0 (pb : alk. paper)
    1. Geriatric nursing--Handbooks, manuals, etc. 2.   Beauty, Personal--Handbooks,
manuals, etc. 3. Older women--Care--Handbooks, manuals, etc. I. Title.
    RC954.T39 2009
    618.97'0231--dc22

                                                        2008039081

British Library Cataloguing in Publication Data
A CIP catalogue record for this book is available from the British Library

ISBN 978 1 84310 973 0

Printed and bound in Great Britain by
Athenaeum Press, Gateshead, Tyne and Wear

This book is dedicated to my mother
Ilene Ruby Hawkes (née Martin)
4/3/1921–25/12/1995

Acknowledgements

My appreciation goes to a team of people who have given their time and support to this book:

Dr Diarmid Ross MBChB, DPH, DTMH, FRACMA; Dr Hugo J. Huygens FRACA, FRCS; Dr Anne Millar MB. MRCP (UK), for important issues relating to skin disorders, nutrition and sun safety (special thanks to Anne for reading and reviewing the book); Janet Upcher through various stages of editing, and proofreading, and her time dedicated to this project; Robin Huygens for proofreading the work in its infancy; Carolyn von Opplen for referencing; Pamela Campbell for her photography and the help in preparing the final manuscript; Stuart Campbell for computer updates and maintenance. Finally, thanks to my photographic models Joyce Boxall, Christine Line, Pamela Campbell, Elizabeth Jacob, Connie Clark and Robert Allanby.

Contents

Disclaimer

This book is a reference work based on the author's own experience. Any techniques and suggestions are to be used solely at the reader's discretion. The herbal remedies, essential oils and medical treatments described in this book are in no way to be considered as a substitute for consultation with a medical practitioner, and should be used in conjunction with approved medical treatment. The author and publisher are not responsible for any harm or damage to a person, no matter how caused, as a result of following any suggestions in this book.

Introduction

This book originates in response to a need to inform consumers and carers of the basic techniques of 'home beauty', in cosmetic application and treatment. These techniques can help prevent harmful treatments and overuse of harmful products, often the cause of skin, fingernail, toenail and hair problems. When such problems arise, poor application of cosmetics and treatments is often overlooked as a possible cause. Many people continue to follow outdated ideas, unaware that they may be causing more harm than the good they had intended.

Over the years, working with beauty therapy treatments, I have been asked many questions by clients, carers and nursing staff about cosmetics, fingernail and facial hair problems. During these years, I have come to specialize in beauty therapy in aged-care, valuing the experience I have gained and which I am now able to share with others. The simple methods described in this book are easily applied by a consumer or carer. The reader is also offered guidelines for the safe application of cosmetic treatments. *The Carer's Cosmetic Handbook* is also especially helpful to the person who relies fully on assistance in everyday hygiene.

In the book's seven chapters I give advice and describe simple procedures including cosmetic application for the face and neck, fingernail and toenail treatments and information on facial hair removal for women. Some of the chapters include a question and answer section incorporating the most frequently asked questions.

Throughout this book I have given more attention to the female than to the male. This is because my experience has been working with women, who are more likely to embrace such services. Many of the problems discussed here will be experienced by men and women alike and both will benefit from most of the treatments prescribed in this book.

Cosmetics

The following information is based on cosmetics in general, however, I give more attention to cosmetics relating to facial skin care and to care of fingernails and toenails, hair removal, sun-protection, some essential oils and herbs. An asterisk symbol will indicate important issues relating to older people and persons in care throughout this book.

What are cosmetics?

Cosmetics

'Cosmetics' are a number of products that are used every day for personal use for hair, on the skin, full body treatments, fingernail and toenail treatments, sun care, dental hygiene, body hair treatment and coloured makeup. A cosmetic product is applied to the skin, hair or body part by either rubbing, folding, stroking, patting, brushing, or spraying. The function of a cosmetic is to cleanse or hydrate skin, beautify or enhance features, promote attractiveness, maintain body hygiene and improve skin texture.

Hope in a bottle

There are many brands of skin care cosmetics on the market, most claiming to have some special ingredient that can reduce wrinkles, banish or hide scars, freckles and other minor skin lesions, improve skin texture, and promising a younger-looking skin and so on. When a moisturizing cream is applied to the skin, a process of hydration takes place. If one hydrates a wrinkled area, moisture fills the gaps between the skin folds, giving the appearance of reduced wrinkles, especially if the cream is applied regularly. Should a consumer stop using the cream, the wrinkles will become noticeable again when the skin begins to dry out. However, continued use of creams and protection from the sun may delay the increase of wrinkles.

The function of a moisturizing cream is to help increase the amount of water in the skin, lubricating it, preventing its natural moisture from escaping, making it less brittle.

Q. *What is the difference between cosmetics made for other skin-types compared to the products made for mature-aged persons?*

A. The cosmetic companies in latter years have come to recognize that marketing for the 'mature-aged' bracket is becoming more lucrative as the 'baby boomer' generation ages and lives longer, leading to an increase in the numbers of older people. It is this generation, as well as the younger generation, that presently patronize the beauty salons and consume large amounts of cosmetic products to a greater extent than earlier generations. The cosmetic companies have taken this opportunity to present to the baby boomer generation special creams for the mature-aged person with all the new 'hype' words such as natural, herbal, organic, hypersensitive, and allergy-resistant. This promises the mature consumer the ability to delay or turn back the ageing process. A cosmetic claimed to be for 'mature skin' usually refers to a cream suitable for dry, dehydrated, sensitive or problem skins. People of all ages can have a number of skin disorders, therefore 'mature-aged' products are not necessarily only used for 'aged' persons.

If a cosmetic is promoted with claims that it can retard ageing or cause any chemical or structural change in the skin, hair, etc., then it is considered a medical product, not a cosmetic. Therefore, it should comply with all the medical product requirements. (For cosmetic claims guidelines, see the list of useful websites at the end of this chapter.)

Q. *What is the difference between expensive and inexpensive products?*

A. The only difference between expensive and inexpensive cosmetics is the marketing and packaging. A 'good' cosmetic is defined as beneficial by the action of its main ingredients and their properties. Benefits include its ability to improve skin texture, its ability to provide sun protection, its capacity to do what it claims and not contain any harsh chemical ingredients causing an allergic reaction or sensitivity.

On some occasions during a treatment I have used a less expensive cream or a sorbolene cream on older clients and clients with skin disorders. This has proved to be more beneficial to the skin than an expensive cosmetic cream.

Cosmetic ingredients

In Australia*, the law requires that all ingredients be identified on the packaging of cosmetic goods sold in Australia. This enables consumers to identify products that contain ingredients which may cause an allergic reaction or be potentially harmful. Understanding cosmetic ingredients is a complex subject and confusing for many consumers. You would possibly need to have a science or chemistry degree to fully comprehend how substances interact

---

*   See the list of useful websites at the end of this chapter for laws governing cosmetic ingredients in United States of America, Australia, Canada, and the United Kingdom.

with each other and living cells. My personal experience in the understanding of cosmetic ingredients is to refer to a cosmetic dictionary or to look up cosmetic ingredients on the internet. Basically what you need to know is product safety; are the ingredients harmless or toxic? What are the side effects? And can its function satisfy its claims?

Q. *Should I be confused when reading the labels on cosmetics?*

A. Yes, most people are. Generally the most important ingredient is listed first, followed by the next important ingredient and so on. The further down the scale, the lesser the effect that ingredient will have. This will give you an idea of the amount of a harmless or toxic ingredient that has been included in the product.

Q. *What are some of the side effects of harmful ingredients?*

A. A person can suffer from a number of side effects at one time with minor or major reactions. Some of the side effects that show are redness, swelling, blistering, weals, hives, sores, lesions, pimples, hair loss, scars, burns, skin peeling and spots. The person may also feel a burning sensation, stinging, nausea, dizziness, headache, and may experience a runny nose, sneezing, coughing and watery eyes.

Q. *How safe are cosmetics?*

A. Before being considered suitable for consumer use, all cosmetics have to pass a certain standard in Australia* set by the Australian Competition and Consumer Commission (under the Trades Act 1974) and the National Industrial Chemical Notification Assessment for labelling of cosmetics. Products must also have warning labels if certain ingredients may cause any harmful side effects. While most people use a number of cosmetics per day and do not experience any harmful side effects, there are many who do suffer the side effects of cosmetics claimed to be harmless. People who have delicate skins, true dry skins, people with an

---

*   See the list of useful websites at the end of this chapter for laws governing the labelling of cosmetic ingredients in United States of America, Australia, Canada, and the United Kingdom.

illness, those on strong medication, older persons and young children are often very vulnerable to the overuse of cosmetics. Cosmetics on the whole need not be the enemy; if they achieve what they claim and try not to break the boundaries of medicine, they can be very valuable. Cosmetics have been used ever since man has roamed the earth, and, to this day, I have never actually heard of anyone dying from an overuse of cosmetics in modern times. However, I have seen major reactions on a few individuals caused by the side effects of harmful ingredients still used in some cosmetics. Cosmetics used correctly and safely can have many benefits and can complement any treatment with excellent results.

Q. *How do I know which cosmetic is right for my client?*

A. If the cosmetic you are using does not give the person any skin problems or cause any stinging or burning, does not feel too greasy, tight, or show a shiny surface, but helps the skin feel and look good, then the cosmetic you are using is probably right. Patch-testing is the best method to determine whether a product is suitable for a particular skin type. (See section on Patch-testing, in this chapter.)

AHAs and RA

Many cosmetics on the market today contain alpha-hydroxy acids (AHAs). Some of these cosmetics contain vitamins in moisturizers, exfoliant creams and lotions.

Q. *What are AHAs and what are the benefits?*

A. AHAs are a group of acids that come from fruits and milk. They are naturally occurring chemicals that help to break down the inter-cellular glue that holds the surface of the skin cells together. The acids that occur in these foods are:

Citric acid (from oranges and lemons)

Glycolic acid (from sugar cane)

Malic acid (from unripened pears and apples)

Mandelic acids (extract of bitter almonds)

Tartaric acid (found in fermented grapes and wine)

Lactic acid (from fermented milk).

These acids are produced synthetically for cosmetic use. The AHAs' primary functions are to help remove the layers of dead cells from the skin's surface. This is the reason why many cosmetic companies add these acids in exfoliating creams and lotions. Through exfoliation, AHAs help stimulate the renewal of cells resulting in a faster cell turnover. They help to remove blackheads, treat clogged pores, smooth fine wrinkles and remove dry surface cells, giving the skin a 'younger-looking' appearance.

Q. *Are AHAs beneficial to all skin types?*

A. Unfortunately not all AHA preparations are as effective as they claim. High concentrations of acids can sometimes result in dry, flaky skin, and skin rashes. Some can cause stinging and the skin to redden (erythema), especially on hypersensitive skin types. Higher concentrations of AHAs still require prescription. AHAs in low concentration are classified as 'cosmetics' which alter only the appearance of the skin's surface, not the structure of the connective tissue.

Q. *How do I choose a cosmetic with the right AHA?*

A. AHAs in some cosmetics will show the excellent results they claim for the skin. Cosmetics that contain the AHAs of glycolic and lactic acids can be more effective for fine wrinkles and for treating dry skin. The concentration of AHAs in most cosmetics for consumer use is at a lower level, between 8 per cent and 10 per cent. Continued use of AHAs in any cosmetics may cause the skin to become sensitive to the sun. Some cosmetic creams and lotions that contain AHAs have a sun protection factor (SPF) included. It is always best to apply a sunscreen after using any product that contains AHAs.

AHAs with low acid concentrations may be suitable for use as an exfoliant cream on the skin of an older person. However, always patch-test first, using with caution a very small amount of cream when working on delicate skins. Cosmetics with AHAs may not be suitable for use on the skin of the hypersensitive or the medically frail.

Q. *What is RA and what are its benefits?*

A. Retinoic acid (RA) is the primary form of vitamin A found in the skin. A deficiency of vitamin A can cause impaired vision, weight loss and dry, red, flaky skin. RA is used to treat acne, photoageing (sun damaged skin) and dark spots and decrease wrinkles. RA is very potent, and due to its side effects it requires a prescription and must be used only under the supervision of a doctor. Some cosmetics may contain 'retinol' or 'retinyl' compounds, which are only imitations of RA and may have very little, if any, effect.

Q. *What are the side effects from using RA?*

A. The skin becomes very red, dry and flaky. When the topical cream is first applied, RA increases skin sensitivity to the sun, cosmetics and perfumes. Even low concentrations of RA can cause problems to the skin and because of its harsh side effects some persons are unable to use it.

Q. *What are the benefits of using vitamins in cosmetic creams?*

A. Vitamin A – retinol in its true form will help accelerate the skin's natural exfoliation process and reduce the appearance of fine lines and wrinkles.

Vitamin B2 – riboflavin is used in cosmetics as an emollient. Nutritionally it would have more value to the skin than in cosmetics.

Vitamin C – ascorbic acid keeps skin tight and smooth. Exposure to sunlight will deplete vitamin C levels. Vitamin C is used in cosmetics as a preservative and antioxidant.

Vitamin D2 – calciferol is used for skin-healing in lubricating creams and lotions. Vitamin D is also absorbed through the skin. Vitamin D from the sun would be more beneficial than in cosmetics.

Vitamin E – tocopherol is obtained from edible vegetable oils. It is used as an antioxidant in cosmetics such as baby creams, deodorants, hair products, moisturizers and cleansers. It is good for wound healing, dry skin and scar tissue. It helps to protect the cell membranes from destruction of environmental pollutants.

Using vitamin E in a cream or sunscreen before going out into the sun will help to protect the skin from dryness, sensitivity and the effects of sunburn.

Q. *What are antioxidants?*

A. Antioxidants are preservatives that prevent fats from spoiling. They can prevent other substances from oxidating such as vitamins A, D, K, E and selenium, all of which are fat-soluble. Vitamin C has antioxidant properties and is water-soluble. Antioxidants are important as they protect the body from poisonous substances.

Q. *What are free radicals?*

A. Free radicals are unstable molecules that are produced by the body as a result of its natural metabolism and as part of its natural defence against disease. Sometimes the body overreacts, increasing free radical production, releasing more of the unstable molecules than it needs. Factors that spark their overproduction are exposure either to the sun or to certain cancer-causing agents in the environment; other factors include illness and smoking. Too many free radicals damage connective tissue, cell membranes and DNA – the basic genetic building block. Premature ageing of the skin and skin cancer can be caused by free radicals. Antioxidants protect cell membranes from free radical damage.

Cosmetic absorption

Q. *Does the skin absorb cosmetics which then find their way into the bloodstream?*

A. The ingredients in a cosmetic product should not penetrate the dermis, a deeper layer of the skin or 'true skin', where they could be absorbed into the blood and lymph and thus travel round the body. This process would make the cosmetic a medical product. However, some cosmetic companies have always promoted their skin-care products beyond the boundaries dividing beauty and medicine. Some ingredients such as alcohol, fats, tiny molecules from essential oils, and petroleum-derived hydrocarbons do enter the dermis, carrying soluble substances with them. However, the amounts from a cosmetic product that reach the blood or lymph are probably too small to have much, if any, effect (Stanway 2000, p.28).

Skin care for the face

Q. *How much moisturizing cream should I put on the face?*

A. A cosmetic cream does not need to be applied to the skin like a medical cream, which is generally applied more liberally. For a cosmetic cream you only need a small amount, or as much as the skin can absorb. More can be added through the day should the skin start to dehydrate. The amount of cream or lotion to be applied to the face would be a small portion, about the size of a thumb nail. For oily skins, I would use less, as lotions for oily skins are usually very thin and spread more easily.

Q. *How many applications of cream should I use daily?*

A. Generally about twice daily for true dry skin, dehydrated to normal skin, and maybe once daily for oily skins. The skin itself produces sebum (oil), the skin's natural moisturizing agent. Too many harsh products used at once on the skin can cause it to become drier and more sensitive as these will strip the skin of its natural moisturizing agent. In some cases it may not be necessary to moisturize a very oily skin each day. However, cleansing of the skin must be carried out daily, no matter what the skin type.

Q. *What are the benefits of using a tinted moisturizer?*

A. Tinted moisturizers are mixed with a touch of coloured foundation and moisturizing cream containing a sun protection factor (SPF) or titanium dioxide (another form of SPF). Tinted moisturizers are worn through the day over a daily moisturizing cream. Tinted moisturizing creams can also be used as a daily moisture cream for oily skins as they are mostly non-oily and are more water-based. Their function is to protect the skin from the sun's rays, giving the complexion a healthy glow. Not only do they look good, but they can act as a substitute for foundation.

Some tinted moisturizers are suitable for all skin types while others are specifically made for a particular skin type.

Q. *What cleansers should I use?*

A. Cleansers are packaged in the form of gels, creams, oils, soap bars and foaming lotions. Foaming lotions and cosmetic soap bars are more suited for use on oily/acne-prone skins. Cream-based cleansers or gels are suitable for sensitive skins. Creams, oils, gels and some foaming lotions are suitable for other types of skin. Only a small amount of cleansing cream or lotion is needed to cleanse the face and remove the dirt. Large amounts of cleansing gels or creams applied to the face are only wasted, being washed away with the water along with your money.

Q. *What are the benefits of toners?*

A. It is not necessary to always use a toner as toners are often alcohol-based. Alcohol strips the natural oils from the skin and can cause dryness and redness. Some toners are alcohol-free and are known as skin fresheners. Fresheners give a feeling of freshness and remove any residue left on the skin. Toners do not actually close pores on the skin but their astringent properties may give the appearance of tightening the pores and making them look smaller. Some toners may play a very small part in affecting the pH level of the skin. However, it is the skin's natural moisturizing agent that plays the major part in the skin's pH levels. People with oily skins would benefit from alcohol-free toners.

After-shave lotions in some brands have alcohol that can cause stinging to the pores once the lotion is applied. Men sensitive to these products would benefit from those that are alcohol-free.

Q. *How do I know what moisturizer to use on a particular skin?*

A. The cream-based moisturizers can be used for normal to dehydrated and true dry skins. These cream-based moisturizers range from a thin to a very thick consistency. The thinner the consistency, the more water-based the cream is. This type of cream is suitable for normal to slightly dry skin types and a combination skin of an oily T-zone with slightly dry cheeks and jaw line. Thicker creams are for dehydrated to truly dry skins, and sometimes for sensitive skins. Night creams often come in a thicker consistency and can be used as a day cream. Moisturizers for oily skins come in lotions, milky or liquid creams, gels and are more water-based. Moisturizers are packaged as creams, liquids, lotions, gels and coloured tints.

Skin care cosmetics which are of a different consistency to women's products are available for male consumers. This is because a man's skin texture is thicker and facial hair is coarser. Moisturizing creams and lotions are also packaged for different skin types.

Q. *How can I tell what type of skin a person has?*

A. Skin types range from normal, dry, oily or a combination of any of the above.

A normal skin has an even distribution of oil and sweat on the surface, referred to as the acid mantle. The pH level of the skin should be 4.5, which is acidic. A pH level of 7 is neutral. The normal skin appearance shows fine, slightly visible pores, resulting from an even oil flow. It has a smooth creamy appearance with a slight pinkish glow on the cheeks. No blemishes are visible. This is known as the 'ideal' skin type. Should any blemishes or marks appear, or any changes in oil secretion occur, the skin would then be referred to as 'normal combination', 'normal to oily' or 'normal to dry'.

A dry skin (known as a 'true dry skin') has no oil flow at all. Visible signs are: no visible pores present, dull appearance due to lack of oil, looks thin, and has a fine porcelain appearance with fine lines. The skin feels and looks tight. The skin becomes flaky due to the accumulation of dead skin cells, caused by the lack of sebum (oil).

Dehydrated skin is often confused with dry skin. The difference between a dry skin and a dehydrated skin is that a true dry skin has a lack of oil where a dehydrated skin lacks moisture. A dehydrated skin can affect the entire face or only particular areas of the face. Any skin type can be affected with dehydration. The visual appearance of a dehydrated skin are fine lines on surface of skin, flaky appearance of dead skin, stretched skin and a dull appearance.

Oily skin has a shiny surface due to the excess oil flow accumulating on the surface of the skin. The skin has enlarged pores the oilier the skin, the larger the pores.

Combination skin is not actually a skin type on its own. The word 'combination' relates to the fact that it is made up of all or some skin types, conditions, disorders or imperfections. It may be two skin types, for example, an oily panel with dry cheeks and jaw line. A large percentage of people have this type of skin. 'Oily panel' refers to the T-zone which includes the forehead, nose and chin areas. The T-zone is the area that secretes the most oil on the face.

If you are not sure what your client's skin type is, I suggest a visit to a beauty therapist who will be able to diagnose the type correctly and advise on how to use cosmetic skin care products. A visit to a salon could save a lot of worry and unnecessary money spent in purchasing the wrong products. If you have in your care someone who is unable to travel, some therapists run a mobile service and are available for home, nursing home and hospital visits. Most salons in Australia are unisex and can cater for males.

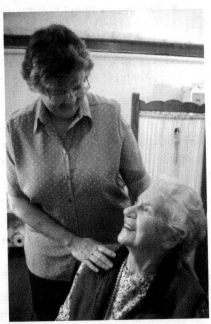

Plate 1.1 The therapist greets her client in the salon. Older women embrace skin care treatments and the use of cosmetic products suitable for their skin.

Sun safe

Q. *Are sunscreens cosmetic?*

A. Sunscreens are classified as 'over-the-counter drugs', not merely cosmetics. This means all ingredients in each preparation have undergone testing to demonstrate their safety and effectiveness. Each particular sunscreen formulation must also be checked prior to sale, to demonstrate its sun protection factor (SPF).

Q. *What sunscreen should I use?*

A. For fair sensitive skin which burns easily, the higher the SPF, the better. People with dark skins would possibly need a lower SPF. This is because the skin has more melanin which protects the skin from the UV rays. However, a sunscreen will help protect the skin from dehydration. The standard SPF range is from 15 to 30[+]. Sunscreen should be waterproof and able to protect the user from UV radiation.

Q. *Why are some people allergic to sunscreens?*

A. As with cosmetics, some people are sensitive to certain ingredients that are used in sunscreens.

If a person becomes sensitive or allergic to any cosmetic or sun cream, you should stop using the offending product and seek medical advice from a doctor or pharmacist.

Herbal cosmetics

Q. *What are the benefits of herbs and essential oils in cosmetics?*

A. These look good on the packaging and encourage the consumer to buy the product by giving the impression that he or she will get the full value of the constituent herbs or oils. In reality, by the time the herbs and oils have been processed and mixed in with other ingredients, their actual function may be very small. During processing, herbs and other cosmetic ingredients lose their natural colouring and therefore without the added colours,

fragrances and preservatives, the cosmetic would be of little value
to a consumer.

Q. *Are home-made cosmetics better to use?*

A. Creating home-made cosmetics can be a lot of fun, by putting
together all natural ingredients without the worry of using synthetic colours and fragrances. They can be of value and very beneficial for the skin and hair. However, just because you are using all
natural products, it does not necessarily mean that a cosmetic will
save certain individuals from having an allergic reaction. Some
natural ingredients in their full natural state can be very harsh to
the skin, more so than their synthetic cousins. Herbs and essential
oils are classified as 'medicinal', and like medication they may
have harmful side-effects and should always be used with caution.
The downside of home-made products is that they have a short
shelf-life and are easily contaminated, as they do not have a
long-lasting preservative to prevent bacteria and fungi from
multiplying.

Patch-testing

When trying a new product, always test with a small amount,
either on the inside of the forearm near the wrist or elbow joint,
jaw line or behind the ears. Leave the cream or lotion for a few
minutes to see if there is a sensitivity, which will produce a
stinging, burning, tingling, hot or cold sensation. If there is an
allergic reaction, the skin will either show redness, redness with
swelling, hives, a rash, red spots or blisters.* Should any of these
signs occur, wash the area with cold water, place a cool compress
over the affected area and wait until the swelling or redness has
ceased. If the affected area spreads and does not settle, seek
medical attention, taking the offending product with you.

---

*   In some individuals, a reaction may only appear after multiple applications. (See skin
     allergies and rashes in Chapter 6)

When I am patch-testing a new product, I generally test it out on willing clients in my salon for a few months before I use it on any person in care. This gives me an idea of how the product has proved its claims, and whether it has produced little, or no, sensitivity or allergic reaction on the majority of those who have had the clinical trials.

As beauty therapists, it is important for us to work with the correct equipment, including the use of cosmetic brands able to live up to their claims and to give satisfactory results. The cosmetic brand should also complement the use of natural products during a treatment. The therapist must be able to use cosmetics that will help to enhance a client's skin, knowing that the cosmetic is 'safe' for a large proportion of clients. Unfortunately, no matter how safe, or how excellently a product is classified, there will always be a few individuals who will have an allergic reaction or a sensitivity to some cosmetic or natural ingredient. Therefore, it is impossible to state that any cosmetic or any 'natural' product is a 100 per cent safe from producing harmful side effects.

Cosmetic hygiene care

Many women of all ages often overlook this most important aspect in maintaining hygiene care in their cosmetics. Lids are either left off jars or tubes, or not put on correctly, leaving the products exposed to the elements. This causes bacteria and fungi to multiply, resulting in contamination. Contaminated products are the cause of many skin problems when a person ignores the signs and continues to use such products, in order to save money. All cosmetics should be used within a limited time, once the product has been opened. Old coloured makeup cosmetics such as foundation, eye shadow palettes, lipsticks, mascara, eye pencils, nail polish should be disposed of regularly, and not kept for years. It will lose its value in colour and texture, and will not enhance the skin as it should when it is fresh and new. Dirty accessories also add to poor application of cosmetics which can spread germs from one area to another.

Many older women and disabled persons are unable to take care of their personal cosmetic hygiene routine due to their physical or mental disability. This task could be taken on by a relative or carer.

Common problems in cosmetics related to the neglect of hygiene

Moisturizers Left exposed to the elements, these become very dry, crack, change colour, and there is sometimes a build up of fungi or dirt as they become badly contaminated. The cosmetic is generally old and should be discarded. Spatulas should be used when taking a product from a container. Using fingers is another way to spread germs from one part of the body to another.

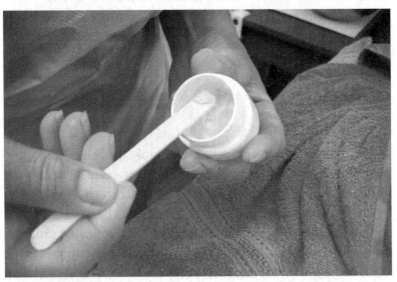

Plate 1.2 Use a disposable spatula to take cream or gel from a cosmetic container.

Compressed powders Stale and left open to the elements, the powder becomes cracked, covered by the unrecognizable powder puff which has been over-used without any cleaning. The dry cracking in the powder is caused by the unclean puff with a build-up of bacteria, sweat and other dirt particles from the person's skin. Cotton pads make a good substitute for a powder puff, as they can be discarded after each use, thus minimizing the build-up of bacteria. The skin should be clean before applying powder.

I personally do not like applying face powder over old stale makeup when the face has been exposed to the elements and dirt has settled on it. Applying more powder traps the dirt and sweat, causing clogging in the skin pores.

Lipsticks The lipstick is generally worked down to the last trace of colour in the tube or container. A build-up of bacteria gathers on the tube as it is exposed to air. Contamination spreads by lending a lipstick to another person, when cold sores can erupt and other lip lesions may occur. Lipsticks should never be shared and should be kept clean at all times. To clean a lipstick colour, scrape the top layer off with a spatula to prevent further spread of contamination, or wipe the lipstick on a tissue. Using a lip brush would help prevent further contamination, provided it is kept clean.

As most frail older women are unable to use a lip brush, a tissue wipe after tube application would be enough to save the build-up of bacteria, provided this is done after each use.

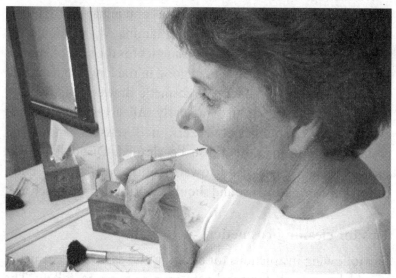

Plate 1.3 The model is applying lipstick with a lip brush. Using a lip brush will help to prevent further spread of contamination, providing the lip brush is kept clean.

Eyebrow pencils Some pencils are very old, worked down to the end, left unsharpened and uncovered, staining the cosmetic bag. Old eye pencils lose colour and texture and should be replaced regularly. Contaminated pencils have a quick way of spreading infections to the eyes.

Do not use old worn-out eye pencils on frail older women.

Nail varnish This is often very old and if left open to the air, will become very thick. The varnish also builds up around the rim of the bottle which makes it more difficult to replace the lid. Nail varnish at this stage should be discarded. To keep the nail varnish bottle and rim clean, use a cotton ball and damp with a non-acetone nail varnish remover. Wipe around the rim of the bottle to remove the build-up of the dry varnish. Clean the brush using a clean cotton ball with nail polish remover before replacing it back into the bottle. Keeping the lid closed tightly on the bottle will delay thickening of the varnish.

Never use thick or old varnish on frail women especially if they are in care. (See Chapter 2 on Fingernail and Toenail Disorders, Manicures and Pedicures.)

When the ingredients of any cosmetic product are exposed to air, or left in moist places, they can become contaminated by bacteria and fungi. Once a product is contaminated, it should be discarded. Continued use of old cosmetics for the sake of 'money saving' can cause more harm than good in the long run, which in turn may cost more money. All cosmetic drawers, shelves, and products should be cleaned regularly. All accessories such as brushes, puffs, sponges, tweezers, nail scissors, and other cosmetic equipment should also be cleaned. Disposable items such as tissues, paper hand towels, cotton pads, cotton buds, cotton balls are easy to use and should be discarded after each use.

Tips for cleaning cosmetics

The following instructions for cleaning and sanitizing cosmetics should be enough for the home user or carer to follow. The method for cleaning instruments such as scissors and tweezers, does not replace any other sanitizing or sterilizing procedures that may be carried out in nursing homes, salons, clinics and hospitals. When purchasing a cleaning agent, the instructions must be followed correctly, as some cleansers can cause an irritation to the skin and dermatitis. Always wear protective gloves when handling any of these products.

Q. *What is the difference between sterilization, disinfection and sanitization?*

A. Sterilization is the killing or removal of all micro-organisms in a material or on an object. The sterilization process ensures that even highly resistant bacterial endospores and fungal spores are killed. Sterilization techniques are very difficult to maintain, as it is impossible to completely sterilize equipment and surfaces in the home, or even in a salon. Sterilization is mainly required for hospital procedures.

Disinfection reduces the number of germs to a level where they pose no danger of disease. Disinfection is effective in a salon (almost like sterilization) except that most disinfectants do not kill spores.

Sanitization is the lowest level of decontamination. It reduces bacteria on implements and equipment. Sanitizing mainly refers to thorough washing with only soap or a detergent. This level of cleaning is suitable for the home user.

Method for cleaning cosmetics

To clean brushes, sponges, combs and other cosmetic accessories, wash in a mild shampoo or soap. Rinse thoroughly after washing, place accessories on a clean paper towel, and cover with another piece of paper towel. Alternatively place them in a glass case or on a clean tray covered with a clean cloth or paper towel and allow to dry in sunlight. (The sun is a natural sterilizer and bleaching agent.) When accessories are dry, place them in a clean container or bag, away from dust and exposure to air. Cosmetic jars, tubes and containers can be wiped over using a clean cloth that has had a mild detergent applied to it. Wipe around the top of the jars where the lid is screwed on, as this is the area where cream often builds up from over-use and neglect. Finish wiping the jars and lids with a dry clean cloth or paper towel.

Eye pencils should be sharpened after each use and kept free from other cosmetic products. Coloured powdered makeup can be cleaned by scraping a thin layer of colour away from the palette, then the container can be wiped clean working away from the colour palette. Place a clean tissue or wax paper over the coloured palette/s.

With tweezers, scissors and other cosmetic equipment it is best to soak them in a sanitizing lotion or a mild disinfectant. After soaking, rinse in hot water, and dry with clean paper towelling or an unused disposable cloth. Next, place the instruments in a small clean bag, separated from other cosmetic accessories.

Another method for cleaning instruments is to place them in boiling water for 15–20 minutes. A clean saucepan with a lid or a clean electric pot can be used. Once instruments are cleaned, remove from saucepan and dry on disposable towelling. Place instruments into a clean unused bag or a clean container with a lid. For hygiene, keep the saucepan or pot separate, for the use of instrument cleaning only.

Useful websites

Australian Government – Department of (1991) Health and Ageing–NICNAS (National Industrial Chemical Notification Assessment) Labelling of Cosmetics
www.nicnas.gov.au/Current_Issues/Cosmetics/cosmetic_guide lines_pdf.pdf

Cosmetic Labelling (2006) Canadian Government. Health Canada. Accessed June 2008 at
www.cbc.ca/news/background/health/labels-cosmetics.html

Cosmetic Labelling and cosmetic safety (2004) United Kingdom. Accessed June 2008
www.bseinquiry.gov.uk/report/volume7/chapter2.htm

Cosmetic Labelling (2006) Federal Food, Drug, and Cosmetics ACT (FD&C ACT) and the Fair Packaging and Labelling ACT (FPLA) United States of America. Accessed June 2008
www.cfsan.fda.gov/~dms/cos-lbl.html

Cancer Australia
www.cancer.org.au/

Sun smart (2008)
www.cancer.org.au/sunsmart

Cancer UK – National Organisations (20/July/2003)
www.cancerindex.org/clink44k.htm

International Nomenclature for Cosmetic Ingredients (INCI) System
www.hc-sc.gc.ca/cps-spc/person/cosmet/ingredients/faq_cons-eng.php

The Australian Competition and Consumer Commission (ACCC)
www.accc.gov.au

Therapeutic Goods Administration (TGA)
www.tga.gov.au/docs/html/cosclaim.htm

Paula's Choice – Cosmetic Ingredients (2007)
www.cosmeticscop.com/cosmetic-ingredient-dictionary.aspx

Glossary

Absorption	The taking in or reception of a substance by skin or tissue.
Accessories	Additional items such as disposable products, cosmetic instruments and utensils.
Added colours	Both natural and synthetic colouring agents.
Allergy	Reaction caused by a substance used externally or taken internally.
Astringent	A substance used to contract tissue by precipitating proteins thus helping to reduce secretions and discharges.
Bacteria	One-celled organisms which multiply rapidly in the right environment.
Beauty therapist	A specialist in beauty culture: able to diagnose skin types and administer treatments relating to beauty care.
Carer	A person responsible for another person's welfare while they are in full or part-time care.
Chemicals	Substances produced by or used in a chemical process.
Collagen	Protein found in connective tissue.
Constituents	Substances forming part of a compound.
Dehydration	Abnormal loss of body water. The deprivation or loss of water from the tissues.
Emollient	An agent that softens and soothes the skin. Used in cosmetics and medicated creams.
Emulsion	The suspension or dispersion of liquid in another liquid.
Exfoliate	To remove dead skin cells from the surface of the skin.

Fungus   A group of eukaryotic organisms found in yeast, moulds and mushrooms and marked by the absence of chlorophyll. Fungus grows in moist, dark areas and is reproduced by spores.

Gum   A mucilaginous secretion of various plants.

Herbal infusion   Plant material infused in warm water.

Herbs   Plants used singularly or in combination for medicinal and other purposes.

High-care   Refers to a person who is unable to take care of themselves being reliant on full-time care by a relative, carer or nurse.

Humectant   A substance used to preserve the moisture content in materials, especially in hand creams and lotions.

Immunity   The body's defence mechanism which fights against the invasion of foreign bodies.

Impurities   Poisons (toxins), foreign bodies, dirt and excrement that invades the body's internal or external environment.

Irradiation   Exposure to radiant energy heat, rays etc. used for therapeutic or diagnostic purposes.

Minerals   In minute quantities minerals are essential components of enzymes that help the body with various chemical reactions.

Preservative   Used in food and cosmetics to prevent contamination and to extend shelf life.

Resin   A solid or semi-solid amorphous organic substance from the sap of plants or can be produced synthetically. Insoluble in water.

Sanitize

To clean and keep bacteria from spreading by the use of mild detergents, soaps, etc.

Sebum

Oily secretions of the sebaceous glands that open into hair follicles.

Skin texture

Identifies the skin's condition, feel and overall look.

Solvent

A liquid capable of dissolving or dispersing one or more substances.

Sorbitan stearate

Used to thicken and stabilize cosmetic formulations.

Sorbitol

A white crystalline powder derived synthetically or from natural sources and used in the manufacture of resins and varnishes and in foods as a sugar substitute.

Therapeutic

Having a curative and relaxing effect.

Titanium dioxide

A mineral salt used as a white pigment in makeup and a physical sunblock in high SPF sunscreen and some cosmetic creams. It has no known external toxicity.

Toluene

A colourless liquid hydrocarbon used in nail varnish. It is obtained from petroleum or by distilling tolu balsam and used mainly as a solvent. May cause mild anaemia if ingested and is narcotic in high concentrations.

Toxins

Poisonous substances which cause tissue destruction.

Ultra violet (UV) rays

Exposure to these accelerates the ageing process and is the main cause of skin cancer melanoma.

CHAPTER 2

Fingernail and Toenail Disorders, Manicures and Pedicures

Fingernail and toenail disorders
Older people in care
Manicures and pedicures
• Manicures for older people in care
• Basic manicure procedure for the home user
Useful websites
Glossary

Fingernail and toenail disorders

Fingernails normally grow about 0.05 to 1.2 millimetres a week (1/8th inch monthly). They tend to grow faster in the spring and summer, with fingernails growing more quickly than toenails. Nails are made up of keratin, protein and sulphur and nail abnormalities often result from nutritional deficiencies. Other problems which can cause nail disorders are medication, illness, infection, external damage and improper manicure or pedicure procedures.

People who rely on manual work for a living are often prone to nail damage and hand problems, due to overuse and lack of daily attention. Musicians, chefs, cooks, gardeners, hairdressers, cleaners, those in the building industry and health care practitioners may suffer with nail deformities, nail disorders, nail damage and hand strain (carpal tunnel syndrome) during their working life.

A healthy set of nails will show a pink colour through the nail plate and the 'half moons' (Lunula) will appear lighter than the rest of the nail because there are fewer blood vessels. The nail plate is smooth and shiny due to the nail's natural oil flow. The nails are strong and the cuticles are firm and smooth. The nail is made up of:

1   **Nail bed** This lies underneath the nail plate.

2   **Nail plate** This is the clear visible part of the nail and the part to buff and varnish.

3   **Free-edge** This is the dead part of the nail which grows above the top of the finger to give it its length.

4   **Cuticle** Skin that protects the nail at the base of the finger, thumb and toes. It protects the skin and nails from infection.

5   **The matrix** This lies underneath the base of the nail and is where nails form from the **nail root** and where they are provided with nutrients from small blood vessels for nail growth.

6   **Half Moon** also called **Lunula** It is live and has fewer blood vessels which give it a light appearance.

7   **Nail fold** This is the skin that surrounds the nail and is prone to split through neglect and is referred to as a 'hang nail'.

Q. *How long should you let nails grow?*

A. To maintain a healthy length of a fingernail, allow the nail to grow above the top of the finger (free-edge), so that when you have the palm of the hand facing you, you can see the top of each nail like the first appearance of the sun coming up behind the mountain. If you cannot see this, the nails may be too short. ('A little bit of length, gives a little bit of strength.') Nails which are too short become weak and cause splitting, flaking and the top layers of the nail plate to shed. The toenails should be a little shorter than the fingernails. If they are too long, footwear can be uncomfortable. Toenails are also stronger and thicker than fingernails.

Short fingernail problems are common among older people, as most would prefer their nails to be very short and will continue to cut them, or have them cut poorly by untrained persons. This leaves the nails open to trauma and infections.

Q. *If nails are stained from smoking, what can I do to improve them?*

A. First of all, encourage the person to, stop smoking. Through smoking, the nails discolour to a yellow or dark yellow, brown hue. The free-edge of the nail becomes black, giving the appearance of dirt in the nails and the surrounding skin of the finger is also affected from the stains. Smoking causes nutritional deficiencies and this shows through the nail plate with deep furrows in the nail, as well as splitting, flaking and weakening. It is not a good idea to use a colour varnish or any clear varnish over the stains to try to cover them up as this can make things worse by weakening the nails further. There are bleaching agents that can help reduce the stains, or a visit to a professional therapist for nail treatment may produce some improvement. However, if the person is going to continue to smoke, the treatments can only be temporary.

Q. *What causes ridges in the nails?*

A. Ridges are also called furrows (little grooves or trenches). In the fingernail, if lines show across the nail plate they are referred to as Beau's Lines. Beau's Lines can be caused by a severe illness, interruption of protein formation, chemotherapy or external damage. Furrows running across a nail plate can also relate to a vitamin or mineral deficiency. Furrows that run lengthways can relate to an injury, smoking, internal disorders, advancing age, or a fungal infection.

Furrows in the nails are common in frail persons with diabetes. Other problems occurring in the nails of a person with diabetes are that the nails can become very thick or very thin and the colour of the nails can appear very pale. Sometimes the nails can have a pale yellowish brown hue which may indicate a kidney imbalance. Infection is another disadvantage due to the dryness in the nails and fingers. Dry skin around the fingers flakes and cracks, the cuticles and nail fold split and this may lead to infection. Once the skin and nails are infected, the person should seek medical advice. A cosmetic hand cream and nail oils may help prevent the skin and nails from drying out, if applied daily.

Q. *How common are fungal infections in the nail?*

A. In my experience, I have found it to be fairly common, especially among frail people. On some occasions I have seen a fungal infection occurring in the feet of a young person who swims and plays sport. Fungal infections can occur in the fingers, fingernails, feet and toenails. In the hands and fingernails, older persons who have suffered a stroke, or have a severe form of arthritis, are prone to fungal infections due to their inability to care for themselves. The affected hand becomes moist and warm due to its lack of mobility. Older people living alone are often prone to a fungal infection in the feet or toenails. This may be due to the fact that they are no longer able to bend over and wipe their feet dry after showering, leaving their feet damp and moist. Circulation is often a problem among older persons, therefore they will feel the cold more (even in warm weather), and will continue to wear stockings or socks and closed-in shoes, leaving little space or time for 'airing' the feet. The warm dark space between feet, stockings, socks and shoes is an ideal place for fungi to grow and multiply. Fungal infections will damage the nail causing it to flake, peel away and fall off. You are not mistaken when you come across a fungal infection in the hands or feet. There is a distinct mouldy, sweet sickly smell and these infections should be treated by a medical person, either a doctor or a nurse.

Q. *What is the cause of a very thick thumbnail?*

A. Sometimes the free-edge of the nail will curve over towards the thumb pad of the thumb, resembling a 'ram's horn' look. It may be the result of a chronic illness, poor blood supply or infection. If all the nails are affected, this may be the result of an internal imbalance, external injury, medication, infection or old age. Never try to cut thick nails; leave this up to the beauty therapists or nail technician. Filing can be an option, if done correctly. (See section on Manicure procedure.)

Q. *What causes ingrowing nails?*

A. Ingrowing nails are more common in the big toes, though they can occur in the fingers as well. Ingrown nails in the fingers are usually caused through improper manicure procedures. In the feet they can be caused through improper footwear, pedicure treatment, or some other trauma. This condition should be seen by a podiatrist or a medical person.

Q. *What causes white spots in the nail?*

A. The white spots showing through the nail plate may be caused by an infection, injury or improper manicure or pedicure procedures. The spots generally grow out with the nail.

Q. *What causes white nails?*

A. This could be due to a lack of protein or anaemia. It may also relate to a liver or kidney disease. White lines across the nail may indicate a liver disorder and white nails with dark spots or streaks at the tip of the nail may relate to a kidney disorder. These conditions should be checked by a medical practitioner.

Q. *What causes hangnails?*

A. The cuticle and surrounding tissue around the nail fold splits which is caused by frequent hand-washing, cutting or biting too close to the cuticles or nail fold. The habit of biting tears away the skin, leaving the area exposed to bacterial infections. Never try to cut too close to the cuticles. It is the dead skin that needs to be shed away from the cuticles and the use of cuticle cream or oil

helps to loosen this dead skin. (See Manicure and pedicure procedure this chapter.)

Q. *What are the signs of a bacterial infection in the nail?*

A. Redness, swelling and pain often indicate a bacterial infection
in the nail or around the nail of the finger or toe. The infection can
turn septic causing pus to accumulate in the affected area. Bacterial infections should be treated by a medical person.

*Frail older people are prone to bacterial infections because of poor
manicure or pedicure treatment, injury and lack of hygienic care of utensils
and cosmetics.*

Q. *What causes nails to be very thin and split all the time?*

A. This condition is referred to as 'egg-shell' nails because of their
thinness, flexibility and tendency to bend and break. The cause
may be due to medication, internal disease, poor diet or a nervous
disorder. Having regular treatments with a nail technician or
beauty therapist and a well balanced diet will help improve this
condition.

Q. *I can't get my nails to grow, as they always split. Why?*

A. Hands immersed in water frequently will cause the free-edge of
the nail to become fragile causing the nail to split and fray. This is
a common problem among many healthcare practitioners. Water
will soften nails and cause drying as it can strip the nail of its
natural oils. To help solve the problem, buff the nails daily and
apply nail oils and hand creams or lotions throughout the day.
(See manicure procedure for the home user this chapter.)

Q. *What are the side effects of constantly using coloured nail varnish?*

A. The on-going use of coloured nail varnish without giving the
nails 'breathing space' can discolour and weaken the nails. This
causes them to split and shed layers of nail tissue from the top of
the nail plate which has accumulated from the build-up of
coloured nail varnish. Some women will apply a fresh coat of
varnish over the old colour left on the nail and this in turn makes
the nail more vulnerable to further damage. To make matters
worse, the varnish in the bottle may be stale or contaminated,

having been exposed to the air, causing thickening, and subsequent difficulty in application.

Nail varnish can induce allergic reactions in sensitive skin, as it holds an ingredient (toluene-sulphonamide-formaldehyde resin[*]) that can cause a rash and a form of dermatitis. Old varnish, coloured or clear, painted on to the nails, should be removed properly with a non-acetone varnish remover before applying any new colour. Nail varnish removers with acetone will strip the nail of its natural oils causing drying and splitting. Varnish removers (with acetone and non-acetone) can also cause a person to sneeze, cough or have difficulty in breathing. Discontinue use of the varnish remover if a person has any of these side effects.

Do not use any varnish, clear or coloured, on a person who is very frail. A medical practitioner may well use the nail bed as a basis to diagnose. It is vital to keep nails clear prior to surgery. This is so that medical staff can check the nails for oxygen levels and the patient's circulation.

Colour showing through the nail plate comes from the nail bed beneath the nail plate, and this can indicate that something may be happening internally. If the trauma or disorder is external, it will show up on top of the nail plate first.

Q. *What can I do, when a resident wants colour varnish applied, knowing that it is not a good idea when the nails are in poor condition?*

A. This is a hard one. I face this dilemma often when working with frail women and forgetful clients. Sometimes it is difficult to make them understand the rationale for non-application of nail varnish. In my case, when I visit the nursing homes, I may have more success when I can rely on the diversional therapist or a carer to remove the varnish after a few days. This allows the nails to have 'breathing space'. Also I can persuade some clients not to have polish on their nails all the time and only have the colour applied to the nails on special occasions. Omitting nail varnish applied to the nails can allow them to regenerate and look better.

---

*   Recently, the ingredient toluene-sulphonamide-formaldehyde has not been included in some of the new nail polishes and these may be an option for use on women in care. However, the downside is that they are expensive and once exposed to the air, the colour varnishes thicken more quickly than those that do contain the offending ingredient.

Perhaps you could have 'resident beauty care days' where you clean and massage the fingers and hands without using varnish, letting the residents know this is 'Hand Care Week' and the following week can be the 'Coloured Nails Day'. Unfortunately, there are some women who are very persistent about having colour applied to their nails. In these cases you do not have much option, as the person has every right to choice. This is where a beauty therapist can be of great help, as their expertise can be very valuable to many older people, especially to those in care.

Older people in care

For frail older people who suffer with an ongoing illness, it is impossible to restore the nails to their original 'health-form' once trauma or damage has occurred. However, I have found among many older clients that there has been an improvement to their nails and prevention from further deterioration when they continue to have regular fingernail care. It is important that people in care should be encouraged to have regular visits from a therapist, as a therapist can bring a 'little something special' to add to their health and well-being. Older people in care look forward to these visits, especially if other visitors are few. Therapists have the time to talk and spend some extra quality time, which is very valuable both to the client and therapist. Because of all the underlying issues related to these people, for example, for those who are diabetic, it is not advisable to give a pedicure treatment, or to cut the toenails. It is best to refer them for podiatry or medical treatment.

Manicures and pedicures

Water is one of the main culprits that can weaken nails and cause the nails to break or fray. Therefore, it is a good idea to file nails before soaking hands and proceeding with a basic manicure procedure. However, when working on the older person in care, soaking the hands first may be a better option because I have found that hard nails are best to file when they are soft, especially hard ram's horn nails and nails with thick furrows. If the nails are very thin as in 'spoon shape' then I would file first before soaking. The following procedures are set out for the carer and home user as a guide to a basic manicure procedure. For the carer's use on the person in care, I will add additional steps denoted by an asterisk.

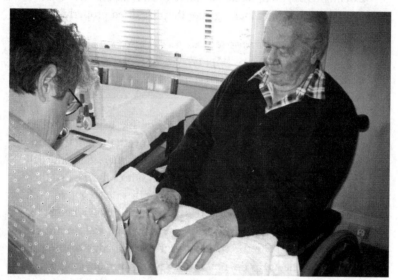

Plate 2.1 The therapist visits a male client in his home. Older men can benefit from a manicure treatment and hand massage.

Manicures for older people in care

A hand roll may be of help when working on a person who has no mobility in their hand/s. To improvise, use a clean face cloth or hand towel. Fold the towel in half then roll the cloth to one end making a hand roll resembling a long sausage. The fingers of the immobile hand can be placed over the roll allowing the fingers to spread making it easier to work on each finger. Another advantage of using a hand roll is to let nail varnish dry while keeping control of the person's hand.

Step one   Remove any old nail varnish from the nails with a cotton ball dipped in a non-acetone varnish remover. Use a separate cotton ball for each finger, hold over the nail for a few seconds and wipe towards the free-edge of the nail. Do this a few times until the entire colour is removed. Repeat as above for all the nails.

Step two   Soak the hands in a bowl of warm water with a cleanser or a drop of essential oil. (See Chapter 3 on Herbal Remedies and Essential Oils.) Soak hands for three to five minutes and remove them from the water making sure they are dried properly.

If the person is unable to immerse hands in water, take a warm wet towel and clean the hands and fingers. Wipe between the fingers as this is the place where moisture builds up and may cause a fungal infection, especially if the person has no mobility in their hands.

Step three   Using a large file (not a metal file which will often cause the nails to fray and split), file underneath the nail horizontally from one corner of the nail across to the other side of the nail until you get an even shape. Use the rough side of the file first then turn over and file the nail with the smooth side to get an even shape. It sometimes may be necessary to cut the nail, whether for convenience or to save time.* Cut across the nail and do not cut corners. You can file the corners from the free-edge of the nail easily. File one way; do not use a sawing motion as this can damage the free-edge of the nail.

Step four   Cuticle cream removers or oils can be applied to the cuticles. Leave for a few minutes to allow time for the cream or oil to soften the dead skin surrounding the cuticle and nail. To remove the dead skin from the base of the nail, use a wooden

---

*   You need to be very careful when cutting across the free-edge on the fingernail of a frail person. Hold your supporting finger across the finger pad of the person receiving treatment and gently move the top of the finger-pad away from the free-edge of the nail, so that the loose skin does not get in the way. The supporting finger also helps prevent any nicks and cuts occurring in the skin. It is best to use nail scissors instead of nail clippers on frail and infirm people. Nail clippers will often tear the nail, especially if the nails are thin, weak, brittle or thick. Breaking the nail can cause more damage and fraying of the nails. Another danger is that it is sometimes difficult to see the nail properly once the nail clipper is over the nail and any loose skin on the finger pad may be caught up and snipped in the process of cutting. Unfortunately I have seen this happen to a few people in care.

cuticle stick and with the flat end gently scrape the dead skin from the base of the nail but not too close to the cuticle itself. Use a tissue to wipe away dead skin after scraping. Do not cut away any skin still attached. Gently push towards the cuticle and leave.

With some older women, I have found that the cuticle skin can grow up towards the free-edge of the nail and sometimes the skin tissue can be difficult to push down. Do not try to push the skin down towards the cuticle if the person feels any soreness or pain. The cuticle nourishing creams or essential oils help shed the dead skin if they are applied every few days. Another condition common in a few frail older people is Pterygium, an abnormal growth of the cuticle skin growing up over the nail plate. This is caused by trauma to the matrix and should be treated by a medical person.

Step five   Using the other end of a cuticle stick, wrap it in a small piece of cotton wool, dip the stick in cuticle oil or some base oil and gently wipe underneath the free-edge of the nail. Use fresh cotton wool at the tip on the cuticle stick for each nail. To remove very stubborn dirt or faecal matter, using an eye dropper with base oil, place a drop of oil beneath each nail and leave for a few minutes. Remove the dirt from each nail with the cotton-tipped cuticle stick or a cotton bud. Once the dirt is removed, soak the hands again. To save time, a resident in care could have the oil applied to the fingernails before shower time and after the shower this would make it easier to remove the dirt. Use a cuticle oil, cream or essential oil to nourish the nails and cuticles and one drop of oil would be sufficient for the treatment of one hand. (See Chapter 3, Herbal Remedies and Essential Oils.)

Step six   Wipe off any excess oil using a tissue or soft buffer to give a shine to the nails. Buffing helps stimulate the natural oil secretions and makes the nails smoother.

---

*   Using a nail brush on a frail person may prove to be very painful for them due to the decrease in the subcutaneous (fatty) tissue beneath the finger and thumb pads. The decrease in fatty tissue and elasticity in the skin will often show the skin to be loose around the finger and nail and the finger appears to be more pointed on some persons. When the fingers have lost their elasticity, I have found many clients have a high sensitivity in their fingers and the nails. (This is possibly another reason why some frail people have difficulty in picking things up because of the tenderness in their fingers or hands.) The fingers are more prone to infection if any slight graze or break in skin tissue occurs, either through scrubbing with a nail brush (even if soft), poor manicure procedures or self-inflicted trauma to the hands and nails.

Step seven   Apply hand lotions, creams or almond base oil to the hands and arms, and massage gently.

Some older women love to have a massage on the arms and hands, as their skin is often very dry. Hand lotion, cream or oil applied with touch is so relaxing and a comfort to them. I have often incorporated hand reflexology in a hand massage that has proved to be successful among many of my older clients. If you are using a new product on a person, do not forget to patch-test first as some individuals may have an allergic reaction or a high sensitivity to the product.

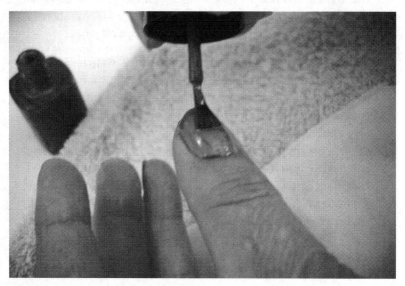

Plate 2.2 Apply a coat of colour varnish to the thumb nail after applying a clear base coat.

There is no need to put any other cosmetic treatment in the 'basic' manicure procedure. If you want to add colour varnish, first coat the nails with a base coat or nail hardener before applying the colour. It is not necessary to apply a top coat as some coloured varnish will incorporate this in with the colour.

Basic manicure procedure for the home user

1 Remove stale polish using a non-acetone nail varnish remover.

2 Apply cuticle remover to the cuticles and leave for a few minutes.

3 File the nails using the rough side of the file starting from the edge of the nail going horizontally across the nail to the other side. Do this several times until you have the shape of the nail and turn the file to the other side using the smooth side for a smooth finish.

4 Soak hands in a bowl using either a herbal infusion, added essential oils to the water, or a foaming cleanser.

5 If the hands are dry, use an exfoliant cream to remove dead skin and soak the hands again. If the nails are still dirty, follow the instruction for Step five in manicure procedure for the older person in care.

6 Scrape away any dead skin from the cuticles using a cuticle stick.

7 Use a white pencil underneath the nails to camouflage stains. This also adds depth to the nails and gives an appearance of the 'French polish'.

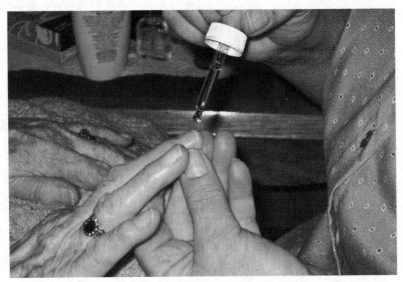

Plate 2.3 Adding essential oils to the nails helps to nourish them and remove dirt. The essential oils have an affinity with the natural nail oils and work well in helping to strengthen the nails and combat infection.

8 Apply the essential nail oils, cream or lotion to the cuticles and nails. Rub into the cuticles, over the nail plate and around the nail fold.

9 Apply hand lotion and massage into the hands, fingers and arms.

10 Buff nails either with a buffer file or rub fingernails together in a criss cross fashion. This helps stimulate the nails' natural oils which help them look clear, healthy and shiny.

11 If you want to wear coloured nail varnish, make sure the nails are completely dry, and then apply a base coat. This helps to prevent the colour of the varnish seeping into the nail plate. Next add two coats of colour making sure the first coat is dry before adding the next coat. If you are

only using a top clear coat, one application should be enough.

A daily routine for nail care (5 minutes maximum)

1   Clean nails (it is best if coloured nail varnish is removed).

2   Apply cuticle strengthening cream or oils to the nails (this will help prevent the cuticles from splitting).

3   Apply hand cream to hands and arms.

4   Buff nails by gently rubbing nails together in a sideways motion, or you can use a smooth buffing brush or file.

This routine can be carried out each day, helping to keep the nails healthy and strong.

Pedicures

A pedicure can be carried out in the same manner as a manicure except it is better to soak the feet in a bowl or foot spa. After soaking the feet, use a pumice stone or foot brush to exfoliate the feet and toes. Wipe feet and toes dry and proceed with the steps used for manicure. The five-minute routine can also be applied to the feet. For buffing, use a smooth buffer file or wipe with a tissue.

Taking care of the nails need not be a difficult task. Daily care can keep the nails in good order and help prevent problems from occurring. Those people at risk from daily manual work would benefit greatly by paying attention to their nails and hands. When I see a musician playing a piano on television it is a pity to see that the pianist has neglected their fingernails and cuticles, and this is emphasized when the camera takes close shots of their hands. The pianist has taken so much trouble to dress and groom themselves, when the most important feature to be on show is the hands. Taking care of the hands is just as important in daily grooming, as neglect can lead to a strain injury, dry skin and infections. So daily nail grooming is not just a 'glamour' procedure for women, it is also beneficial to men and is considered as 'holistic care'.

Visiting a nail technician or beauty therapist is money well spent. It can save you a lot of time and worry in the long run, maintaining hygiene, healthy skin, and promoting education in self-help.

Useful websites

The website listed below was current at the time of writing (30 June 2008).

Dr Loretta J. Standley (2008). Nail Disorders
www.drstandley.com/naildisorders_index.shtml

Glossary

Acetone	A solvent used mainly in nail varnish and nail polish removers. It is an irritant and its use in cosmetics has been banned or restricted in many countries.
Arthritis	An inflammatory or degenerative change which can affect all joints in the body.
Base oils	Vegetable oils used with essential oils and as ingredients in cosmetics.
Bleach	A strong chemical process or whitening in natural sunlight.
Callus	A horny layer of the epidermis (top layer of skin) due to pressure or friction.
Chronic	Long term.
Compress	Square of gauze used with application of pressure.

Corn	A thickening of the stratum corneum which causes severe pain from pressure on the nerve endings in the corium.
Essential oils	Liquid aromatic components taken from parts of plants.
Formaldehyde	An anti-microbial substance used in many product groups. It is irritating to mucous membranes and can be very toxic. It preserves tissue by killing microbes.
Hyponychium	The top part of the skin between the nail plate and nail bed.
Infection	Invasion of harmful micro-organisms in body tissue.
Infirm	Weak, feeble as from disease or old age.
Lesion	Damaged tissue.
Leukonychia	White nails. Abnormal whiteness of the fingernails or toenails as in spots, streaks or total whiteness.
Matrix	Cell forming area. The base of the fingernail or toenail where the structure of the nail grows.
Medication	Administration of remedies.
Nail technician	A therapist who specializes in fingernail treatment and fingernail art.
Onychauxis	Overgrown nail.
Onychia	Inflammation of the matrix and nail bed.
Onychocryptosis	Ingrown toenail or fingernail.
Onychogryphosis	Ram's horn nail (thick thumbnail or toenail).
Onycholysis	Psoriasis in the fingernails.
Onychomycosis	Fungus-infected nails.
Onychophagia	Bitten nails.

Paronychia	A bacterial infection around the nail plate of the finger or toe.
Pathogens	Germs.
Protein	A complex molecule made from amino acids. Protein is found in animals and plants and can be made by the body, being essential for body growth and repair.
Pterygium	Abnormal growth of the cuticle over the nail plate caused by trauma to the matrix.
Translucent	Clear.
Varnish	Nail colour and clear varnish used to make the fingernails and toenails attractive.
Welfare	Consideration given to the health and well-being of a person.

CHAPTER 3

Herbal Remedies and Essential Oils

Herbs and essential oils*

Many plant species have medicinal properties that are used in both herbal and conventional medicines. They contain active constituents which directly affect the body. These medicinal herbs provide assistance in combating illness and support the body's efforts to regain good health. Herbs are used as

---

* Should any person in care be using a topical medicated cream, it would be best to seek medical advice before using any herbal or essential oil for treatment.

anti-inflammatories, diuretics, laxatives and diaphoretics helping to detoxify the body. Herbal preparations have great value when used in a programme of self-care preventative medicine. They are made up as infusions, decoctions, tinctures, poultices, compresses, capsules or tablets. The herbal plant materials used are leaves, flowers, petals, roots, bulbs, bark, gum resin, rinds, seeds and rhizomes.

Essential oils are natural volatile substances of aromatic plants and trees. They are deposited in specialized tissues in different parts of the plant, its petals, leaves, roots, grass, heartwood, rind, seeds, rhizomes and gum resin. Some essential oils (used on their own) are too highly concentrated for direct use on the skin. They are diluted with a base oil to make them gentler and yet still provide a useful therapeutic effect. Base oils are vegetable, nut or seed oils, many of which, themselves, also have therapeutic properties.

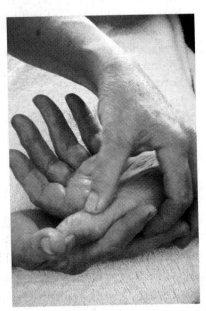

Plate 3.1 Hand reflexology is popular among older people and can be included in a manicure procedure or a massage.

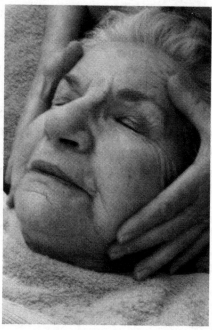

Plate 3.2 Face reflexology can be included in a facial and face massage. Face reflexology helps to improve skin texture and circulation, relieve head tension, headache, stress, sinus problems and it helps to induce sleep. This is a wonderful relaxing therapy for many older persons and persons in care.

I have selected a few of my favourite essential oils and herbs which I use for facial treatment, face reflexology, hand reflexology and fingernail and toenail treatments. I have found these herbs and oils work well with cosmetic treatments and some have proved gentle on the skin without any harsh side effects. This result is good when treating frail, older and infirm people. As mentioned, herbs and essential oils are classified as 'medicines', and must therefore be used with caution. Don't take it for granted that a certain herb will be suitable for everyone. There will always be a certain individual who will show a slight allergic or sensitive reaction, no matter how mild the product may be. Always patch-test when using a herb or essential oil for the first time, especially if using it on a frail or infirm person. To patch-test with herbs, make a herbal infusion. Allow the infusion to cool, and then place a compress over the area of the skin to see if any reaction occurs. With essential oils, patch-testing would be the same as for cosmetics. (See Chapter 1, Cosmetics.)

I have found over the years, while working with essential oils and herbal infusions, the secret is to 'keep it simple'. There is no need to try to add too many oils or herbs together for a particular treatment. One or two oils mixed with base oil and one herbal infusion would adequately treat any skin condition. It takes a lot of skill and understanding to become familiar with the use of herbs and essential oils. For the consumer and carer, I recommend further reading on these subjects. (See the useful websites at the end of this chapter and Chevalier (2001) listed in the Bibliography)

Herbal infusions

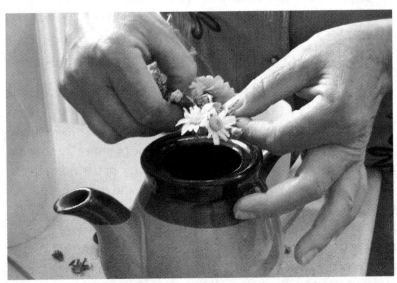

Plate 3.3 Making a herbal infusion using fresh herbs chamomile and marigold

Herbal infusions are made by putting the herb part (leaf, flower, petals and rind) into off-boiling water. Allow to cool before use. Use a china, porcelain, ceramic or pottery teapot letting the herbal constituents seep into the water. An infusion has a short shelf-life and can turn rancid quickly; two to three days in a fridge would be the limit. Once the infusion becomes cloudy, it should be discarded. Infusions are best made daily.

The following are some simple traditional herbal infusion recipes which I find easy to make up for everyday use.

Recipe for a herbal infusion

1 teaspoon of dried herb *or* 3 teaspoons of fresh herb
1 cup of hot water

When I use a herbal infusion on older people in care, I use half the quantity and may add extra water. A mild strength is enough for the infusion to work and not be overpowering to the senses.

For older people in care (or the hypersensitive)

½ teaspoon of dried herb *or* 1½ teaspoons of fresh herb
1 to 1½ cups of hot water

You can dilute the infusion with extra water if the infusion, such as thyme and lavender, is too strong.

Herbal cooling sprays

Herbal infusions make a wonderful cooling spray for warm days. Place the cooling infusion in a cosmetic spray-bottle and spray over the face or part of the body. Keep the spray bottle cool in the fridge. Lavender, peppermint, rose, lemon and calendula (to calm redness in the skin), have a refreshing effect.

Herbal infusions can be frozen into ice-cubes and used as a compress for inflammation, swelling and pain-relief. Marigold and chamomile mixed together are beneficial for ice-cube treatment.

My favourite herbs to use

Aloe (*Aloe vera*. **Family:** *Liliacea*) (Lily family) The gel from its leaf is well known for its properties in healing wounds, burns, sores and scars; it acts as an emollient on the skin. Aloe Vera is used commercially in many cosmetic products. The gel of this herb has a very soothing and cooling effect. I have found that using a little gel on the area of the skin just after waxing helps to minimize any stinging, pain or redness; it also helps while hair is being removed with tweezers.

Chamomile (*Chamomilla matricaria recutita*. **Family:** *Asteraceae*) (Daisy family) Chamomile has anti-inflammatory, anti-allergenic, carminative properties. I love the smell of this herb and not only is it wonderful to drink as a tea, it helps soothe and relax sore eyes. I use this herb as a skin freshener for sensitive and troubled skins. It gives a calming effect and helps prevent, or minimize, any redness of the skin. During a mask treatment I will apply chamomile compress pads to soothe tired and sore eyes. This proves successful for many grateful clients.

Lavender (*Lavandula officinalis syn, Lavandula augustifolia*. **Family:** *Lamiaceae*) (Mint family) Lavender has anti-inflammatory, antiseptic, antibacterial, antioxidant properties. This herb is a favourite among many people of all ages. Lavender is used cosmetically as a skin freshener for oily acne-troubled skin due to its properties of combating bacteria. Lavender scent is very strong and a few individuals may find it overpowering. The constituents in lavender can produce an allergic reaction in hypersensitive skins. I will use the herbal infusion of lavender for oily skins, skin with acne and in a foot spa before a pedicure, or foot reflexology. Lavender is also beneficial for soaking the hands and fingers before a manicure. People who work in the garden and on building sites will benefit from soaking their hands or feet in a lavender infusion.

Lemon[*] (*Citrus limon.* **Family:** *Rutaceae*) (Citrus family) Lemon has antiseptic, antibacterial, antioxidant properties. Lemon acts as a good cleaning agent; therefore I have found the juice helpful for using in a hand wash or soaking hands before a manicure.

Lemon Balm^{**} (*Melissa officinalis.* **Family:** *Lamiaceae*) (Mint family) Lemon balm is a relaxant and has carminative and antiviral properties. Cosmetically it is valuable as a skin freshener for acne-prone skins due to its antibacterial properties. Lemon balm helps relieve cold sores by the use of a compress over the affected area. It can have a slight tingling to stinging effect on the hypersensitive skin.

Marigold (*Calendula officinalis.* **Family:** *Asteraceae*) (Daisy family) This herb has anti-inflammatory, astringent, antiseptic properties. It helps to heal wounds, swelling and redness in the skin. Therefore it is very good for soothing areas of inflammation. This is one herb I can use with ease, as I have found over the years it does not produce any harmful side effects even on the hyper-sensitive skin. After waxing procedures, I have used a marigold infusion as a compress to the waxed area to help minimize redness. I have found using the calendula oils directly on the skin after waxing is also effective.

Thyme (*Thymus vulgaris.* **Family:** *Lamiaceae*) (Mint family) Thyme has antiseptic, antioxidant properties. Cosmetically it can be used as a skin freshener and cleanser. Thyme is not recommended for use if you have high blood pressure or suffer from epilepsy. I have found thyme infusion a beneficial gargle for sore throats, mouth ulcers, or bad breath. This herb works well in relieving soreness in the mouth, throat and gums.

---

*   I do not use lemon on frail people, as the acid in the fruit is too strong and can cause stinging in the surrounding tissue of the fingers.

**   I do not use lemon balm on frail clients.

Dentures soaked in a mild thyme infusion may give relief to the gums when the dentures are placed back in the mouth after soaking. The infusion will also help combat any contamination in the water while soaking the dentures. The dentures must be rinsed after soaking before placing them back in the mouth. Thyme infusion, even though mild, can be strong for some people. I do not use this herb on the skin of frail older people.

Quality control of herbs and oils

Making the most of herbal medicine means ensuring that the herbs and herbal products are of good quality, properly grown, well dried, correctly processed and within their use-by date. Using poor-quality herbal products is all too often a waste of money since they are highly unlikely to be of any benefit. When it comes to herbal medicine, quality is everything. Herbs should be stored in a dark place away from sunlight, which causes oxidation, and affects their efficiency. Good quality aromatic herbs should have a distinct scent and smell. Essential oils and base oils must also be stored away from sunlight. The oils are best kept in the dark bottles in which they are sold. Once oil turns rancid, it will have a sickly smelling stale-fatty odour. Discard out-of-date oils, if they show the slightest change in appearance and smell.

Essential oils and base oils

There are many essential oils with a wide range of fragrances. All of them have special properties and a specific function. I have found over the years, that it is best to stay with some of my favourites and 'keep it simple' especially when working with older people. The home user and carer will benefit from the use of some of the essential oil recipes for fingernail and toenail treatments.

When I work with frail clients, I use essential oils very sparingly due to the many underlying problems they may have in the skin and nails. I would use about one drop of oil diluted with the base oil, just enough for the client to enjoy a familiar smell without feeling overpowered by the fragrance. If the client has a chronic skin problem, they may be using a medicated cream; in this case, medical permission should be sought. In some cases where multiple skin-disorders are visible, it may be all right to use a small amount of base oil without the use of the essential oil, this will still give some positive effect on the skin.

Base oils

There are three main base oils I like to use for skin treatment.

Almond (*Prunis amygdalus* **or** *Amygdalus communis.* **Family:** *Rosaceae***)** Almond oil comes from the kernel of the nut. This is my favourite base oil. It has many valued properties such as vitamins, minerals, protein and glucosides. Almond oil helps to relieve itching, soreness, dryness, inflammation, eczema, dry and dehydrated skins.

This is the base oil I would mostly use on the skins of older persons and for the hypersensitive. This base oil is also used in nail treatments.

Avocado pear oil (*Persea americana.* **Family:** *Lauraceae***)** (Laurel family) The oil comes from the fruit. This oil is good for all skin types. It contains vitamins, protein, lecithin, fatty acids and is good for eczema and troubled skins.

Jojoba oil (*Simmondsia chinensis.* **Family:** *Simmondsiaceae***)** The oil is taken from the bean. Jojoba contains protein, minerals and a waxy substance that mimics collagen. It is widely used in cosmetics, good for inflamed skins, psoriasis, eczema, acne, hair care and all skin types. I find it has value mixed with other oils used for the treatment of nails.

Essential oils for the skin

Lavender Good for calming, relieves muscle pain, stimulates blood flow and helps acne-prone skin.

Marigold Good for wound-healing, acne, boils, tinea, bites, stings, inflammation, varicose veins. (Use for the frail and hyper-sensitive.)

Chamomile Good for inflammation, relaxing, insomnia, stomach upsets, and soothing for eyes. (Use for older people.)

Neroli (*Citrus aurantium*. **Family:** *Rutaceae*) (Citrus family) Neroli are volatile oils from the flowers of bitter orange. The oils are beneficial for stress-related illness and insomnia. It can be used as a gentle sedative and improves skin elasticity. (Use for older people.)

Evening Primrose oil (*Oenothra biennis*. **Family:** *Onagraceae*) Evening Primrose oil is rich in essential fatty acids. It is beneficial for eczema, chapped skin and itchy dry skin.

Sandalwood (*Santalum album*. **Family:** *Santalaceae*) Good for dry skin and sore throats, itchy skin conditions such as Seborrheic dermatitis and contact dermatitis. Recently it has been used for other inflammatory conditions such as for rheumatoid arthritis.

Essential and base oils for the fingernails and toenails

Almond (See above)

Carrot (*Daucus carota*. **Family:** *Umbelliferae*) (Parsley family) Carrot oil contains vitamins, minerals and beta-carotene. Good for the skin and nail treatment. Helps reduce scarring.

Jojoba (See above)

Lavender (See above)

Lemon Has antiseptic, antibacterial and astringent properties. Good for nail care.

Marigold (Calendula) (See above)

Tea-tree (*Melaleuca alternifolia.* **Family:** *Myrtaceae*) (Eucalyptus family) Tea-tree has antibacterial, antifungal and antiviral properties. Good for fungal and bacterial infections. This oil is very strong and should be diluted with base oil*. It can have a burning effect on the skin if used without water or base oil, especially on sensitive skins.

Essential oils as a fragrance

Essential oils make a wonderful substitute for a fragrant perfume, especially if you are allergic to cosmetic perfumes. Many people are unable to wear a strong fragrance for this reason. Some frail older women cannot tolerate the odour of a strong perfume, and can actually have a reaction from the perfume that another person is wearing. This is one of the reasons I do not wear a perfume when visiting clients in their homes or in a nursing home. (The worst smell to me and to some of my clients is when fragrance is used to try and combat the fumes of cigarettes. Unfortunately this makes the smell more repugnant. The chemicals from the cigarettes and perfumes do not mix well together, giving off a strong musty, sickly odour.)

Essential oils can be used as a spray using two or three drops of oil diluted in warm water. Allow to cool before use. (You need to shake the bottle before use, as the oil will separate from the water.) This method has proven successful for many women who

---

* I do not use tea-tree oil on the skin of frail people. Tea-tree oil is best diluted in water and used as a cleanser for soaking hands.

are unable to use commercial cosmetic perfumes. If using a spray-oil on a frail person or a person with a sensitive skin, use one drop of oil to test the fragrance as some oils have strong odours which can be overpowering.

Application of oils for nail treatment

One drop of nail oil from an eye dropper would be enough to gently work the oil in to each finger and thumb of the hand (or possibly both hands) and the same would apply for toes.

For the removal of dead skin around the cuticle area:

Step one   Use a cuticle stick with the flat end wrapped in a tiny piece of cotton wool.

Step two   Place the oil from an eye dropper onto the cuticle stick then brush across the cuticle area, leave for a few minutes, and the dead skin should be easy to scrape away.

Step three   To clean underneath the free-edge of the nail and around the nail, hold an eye dropper under the free-edge, place one small drop of oil on each finger or thumb and allow the oil to run down into the nail, around the sides of the nail and top of the nail plate. Leave for a few minutes and the dirt matter will be easy to remove. This method will also work for those green-fingered people who love to work in the garden.

Oil mixtures for nail treatment

Treatment to help strengthen the nails and cuticles:

> 2 tbs almond base oil
> 3 drops jojoba base oil
> 1 drop sandalwood oil
> 1 drop lavender oil
> 1 drop lemon oil
> 1 drop carrot oil
> 1 drop calendula oil

Treatment to help combat infections:

> 2 tbs almond base oil
> 3 drops jojoba base oil
> 1 drop lemon oil
> 1 drop tea-tree oil
> 1 drop lavender oil (omit if allergic)
> 1 drop calendula oil

For the frail and the sensitive, I would use half the quantity of each essential oil ingredient (e.g. 2 tbs almond oil, 1½ drops of jojoba oil, ½ drop of each essential oil). I would also use the almond, jojoba and just two different essential oils, which should be enough to produce a satisfactory result. The mixture should last a few weeks if the treatment is carried out regularly. Mix oils together in a dark bottle and place away from sunlight.

There are many other essential oil treatments for the nails but the ones I have selected have worked well over the years on many older clients. It would possibly be expensive for the home user to go out and purchase all the oils separately. Using base oil and two different types of essential oils would still be beneficial to the nails. The other alternative is to have the nail treatment mixture made up by your local aromatherapist or a pharmacist who may sell 'ready made' formulas.

Formula for clay mask

Herbal infusions and essential oils combine well with a natural clay to make a face mask. Over the years, I have discovered the benefits from using such a combination, especially for deep cleansing of the pores in the skin.

> 2 heaped teaspoons clay
> 1 drop essential oil (or base oil for sensitive skin)
> 1–2 teaspoon/s of herbal infusion

Place clay in a bowl, add essential oil, pour in the infusion and mix to a paste. The mask should be easy to spread and be enough for the face and neck. Do not spread mixture near eyes or mouth and do not cover nostrils. Lie down and place two cotton pads that have been soaked in a chamomile infusion over the eyes. Relax until the clay has dried. Remove the clay with a warm damp cloth or face washer. Apply a moisture cream to the face after treatment.

Coloured clays can be purchased through small business houses such as pharmacists and health food stores that stock natural products.

Useful websites

The websites listed below are current at the time of my research on 30th June 2008 before publication.

Medicinal (12/2/08): an internet resource on medicinal herbs. www.emedicinal.com

Mrs Grieve's (12/6/08): Botanical names of herbs. www.botanical.com

Botanical and common name of herbs. www.ageless.co.za/herb-jojoba.htm

Glossary

Alternative medicine   Also known as complementary, holistic or natural medicine. Alternative medicine refers to any natural therapy or medicine practised outside the mainstream of western medicine.

Antibacterial	Medicines, detergents, cosmetics that have a constituent able to combat bacterial infections.
Antidepressant	Medicines, natural or western, that can help alleviate depression and calm the nerves.
Antifungal	An agent having the ability to inhibit the spread of fungi.
Anti-inflammatory	Medicines, herbs, cosmetics that can help alleviate inflammation.
Antiviral	An agent that inhibits the proliferation of viruses.
Beta carotene	Pro-vitamin A. Found in all plants and many animal tissue. Used as a colouring in cosmetics.
Carotenoids	The red, yellow and orange pigments found in plants.
Fatty acids	Structural components of fat.
Interstitial fluid	A liquid surrounding all body cells.
Lecithin	Obtained from egg yolk and soybeans. A natural antioxidant and emollient used in cosmetics. Non toxic.
Organic	Denoting natural minerals, plants and materials.
Oxidation	A process essential for survival.
Rancid	Contaminated product giving off a musty sickly smell or stale fatty taste.
Rhizomes	Root-like subterranean stem, commonly horizontal, which produces roots below and sends up shoots from the upper surface.
Virus	Minute infectious agents which invade cells, where they grow and reproduce.

CHAPTER 4

Hair Removal Methods for Women

Hair removal methods
Waxing contraindications
Waxing for older women
Facial hair disorders
The eyebrows
Steps to shaping the eyebrows
Useful websites
Glossary

Hair removal methods

Unwanted hair growth has always been a problem for every age group but methods of hair removal have equally been problematic. Dealing with facial hair in particular, among older women, has caused embarrassment and discomfort. Areas on the face that can be affected by unsightly hair growth are the sides of the face, the chin, top lip and neck. Some methods used to remove hair have caused unnecessary problems, due to lack of skill and to the use of inappropriate products. In the past, some products have been too harsh containing strong chemical substances which cause skin problems and encourage further re-growth of coarse hair. Some of the products on the market today have improved and there are different forms of waxes, creams, gels and sugars to remove unwanted hair. Other forms of hair removal for the home user are shaving, bleaching, epilators and tweezing.

Having hair removed from parts of the body is a personal choice. To one person, the extra re-growth of hair is not a problem, while to another, it can be very stressful. Also, some women can feel uncomfortable having excess chin hair, while hair on the top lip does not concern them. In some cases, women in care do not worry about unsightly facial hair and it is more of a problem to the person who may be the carer or a relative. Unfortunately, some older women who are fully dependant and in care have been shaved by the carer or relative because of this. This is where problems often begin. Shaving should not be used as an alternative on the skin of a frail person. If the woman is happy the way she is, then let things be. Should she want her facial hair removed, employ a therapist who is skilled in hair removal. Waxing on the skin of a frail woman in care should be left to an aesthetician or beauty therapist.

In this chapter, I do not intend to teach the reader waxing procedures as this is a skilled art, and should be used with caution. However, there are many products on the market which the home user can use, providing instructions are clearly understood and followed and hygiene procedures are carried out.

Q. *Why does shaving cause ingrown hairs?*

A. Shaving is the most common method of hair removal for the home user as it is convenient, simple and easy. There are several disadvantages in shaving, especially in areas of the body that are exposed (the face, arms, legs). Shaving only removes hair topically and hair re-growth is rapid. The hairs are strong and coarse and the stubble can feel uncomfortable, especially on the legs. In sensitive areas, such as the bikini line, underarms and face, papules (bumps or blind pimples) can occur. This is because the end of the hair in the follicle is cut off bluntly. The blunt edge of the hair has to force itself through a fine pore which is designed for the tip of very fine hair. Blunt hair pushing through a fine pore can cause irritation in the form of a papule. Another problem with shaving is that, in some cases, the fine pieces of cut hair fall back into the follicle causing an infection in the form of a pustule (pimple). If a hair strand grows out of the follicle and curls back into the skin, this is an ingrowing hair.

Older women with sensitive skins and skin disorders can find shaving irritating, causing further damage. Shaving not only removes hair, it removes dead skin cells breaking down the skin barrier, causing skin sensitivity. Facial shaving can cause the hairs to become strong and coarse, encouraging re-growth. Shaving the face regularly will encourage the hairs of the face to grow thick like a man's beard. When the facial hair has reached this stage in an elderly person, there is, however, not much alternative for removing the unsightly hair. To do so would prove very painful and possibly cause more traumas to the skin.

Q. *What are the benefits of hair-removing creams?*

A. Hair-removing creams are referred to as depilatory creams or gels. They are chemical depilators which remove hair from the skin's surface when the solution is washed away. This method of hair removal results in rapid skin irritation and skin sensitivity. If a chemical solution can dissolve hard keratin in hair, it would prove too strong for use on the average skin. Other problems that some depilatory creams can cause are scarring, burning, rashes and cysts. There are some depilatory creams and gels lately on the market that have less irritating ingredients, however, the removal of hair by a depilatory method can have contraindications for sensitive skins.

Some older women have used these creams most of their adult lives, and through the removal of hair by this method have encountered certain skin problems, such as follicle damage, scarring, hard lumps and a coarse re-growth of hair. The hair re-growth is generally white, and hard to remove.

Q. *What causes the white hairs to grow with the re-growth of facial hair?*

A. Melanocytes located in the basal (bottom layer) of the skin produce the pigment melanin. Melanin in the hair root creates the dark colour of the hair. As we age, melanin stops being produced. The first sign of this happening is when the hair first turns grey, and when the hair is white the body is no longer producing melanin. External damage to the follicle can interfere with the production of melanin, producing white strands of hair mixed in with other natural hair colours. External damage to a hair follicle can be caused through the use of depilatory creams, shaving, improper tweezing or an injury.

Q. *What causes hairs to grow on the face?*

A. On our faces there are fine downy hairs which are light, soft and not so noticeable. However, an internal disorder, such as illness, hormonal changes, intake of certain medications or smoking can make the fine hairs of the face become thick, coarse, brittle, coloured and unsightly. External damage such as injury or improper hair removal may cause the regrowth of coarse hair.

Q. *How is waxing better than the other two methods?*

A. Waxing removes the hair below the skin level, taking the hair bulb with each strand of hair, making it more successful due to its long-lasting effect. The hairs grow back softer and waxing does not affect the skin barrier when skin cells are removed. Over a period of time, the hairs grow back very thin and in some cases, parts of the body cease to reproduce the re-growth of hair.

The downside of waxing is that it can be painful on sensitive skins, and this process may not be suitable for some women.

Q. *What are the best waxing products to use at home?*

A. For the home user, it can be very confusing to sort out which product is best to use when there are various forms of wax on the market. Waxes sold to the home user are packaged in jars, packets and bottles. Waxes in jars are usually cold waxes, or waxes that can be heated up in a microwave oven or hot water. The cold waxes are often sticky and messy and not suitable for use in cold climates as they go very hard. I have also found them to be unreliable in removing the hairs from the hair follicle in one sweep with the cloth. Waxes warmed in the microwave oven have a better effect than cold waxes. However, once again they can be very messy to use. The best waxes I have found are the clear strip waxes which are packaged in boxes. Each strip of wax is held between cellophane paper. The paper strips are pulled apart and both sides of the waxed strip can be used to remove the hair. One can cut the size and shape needed. It is quick and much easier to use than the other waxes. It is more hygienic as it is used once and disposed of after use. The disadvantage is that it can become very sticky, especially in hot weather. Also, if used incorrectly, it can cause irritation to sensitive skins.

I have found using clear wax strips a better alternative for use on the skin of frail women, especially for those who are in care. The hot waxes used in salons and those made for the home user are not an option because of safety and hygiene concerns. Also hot wax on sensitive and thin skins can cause burning and soreness. The advantages of using a strip wax are that I can cut the wax strip to the size I need and at the same time be able to see the amount of hair that is to be removed. Not all older women are sensitive to waxing; many can cope and put up with the short discomfort of the hair being removed for the positive gains. Some clients have commented 'waxing my face is nothing compared to the pain I feel in my body'.

Q. *Why does the skin go red after tweezing or waxing?*

A. Redness of the skin (erythema) is caused by engorgement of capillaries in the lower layers of the skin and occurs with a skin injury, infection or inflammation. After waxing, there is always some form of redness, and this may be due to the hair being pulled out with its bulb attached to the follicle. When the bulbous hair is detached from the follicle, blood fills the empty space, causing the redness and sometimes a tiny droplet of blood to appear on the surface of the skin. Blood will often appear when terminal strong coarse hair has been removed. Waxing over a period of time will cause the hairs to become very thin and sparse and very little or no redness will show, except for those with sensitive skin where inflammation will often recur.

Marigold infusion will help minimize any inflammation and is good to use as a cold compress after waxing. Aloe Vera also soothes the skin of the face, bikini and underarm areas. Baking soda mixed with water can also help with inflammation or with any pustules that occur from waxing. Waxing can cause an over-stimulation of the oil glands, producing pustules or blistering on sensitive and on very oily skins. Cold compresses and ice cubes will also help minimize this problem.

Q. *How often should I wax?*

A. This depends on the individual. Generally for the leg, bikini, and underarm waxing, the re-growth of hair can take up to six weeks or even longer. On the face, waxing can be done any time between two to six weeks, depending on any internal disorder that the person may have. The hairs need to be long enough (about the size of a small fingernail) for them to adhere to the wax and be pulled from the follicle without breaking or splitting. Short hairs are hard to wax and will require tweezing.

Waxing contraindications

Wax treatments may not be suitable for some people, especially those who cannot cope with pain, or who have very sensitive skins, skin disorders, skin infections, high blood pressure, diabetes, oedema, or skin cancers. Failure to follow these warnings may lead to skin irritation, burning, skin removal of the epidermis or other injuries.

Waxing for older women

Age, illness, nutritional impairment, hormonal changes and medication can be the cause of coarse or excess facial hair growth in frail older women. Some medications can cause the hairs to grow thick and coarse, or reduce hair growth in the eyebrows. Age affects the growth of hair which also can be hereditary. An older person's skin becomes loose, sensitive and sometimes may show multiple skin disorders, all of which can make waxing or other forms of hair removal difficult. For diabetics, waxing must be carried out with caution. Because of the slow healing from any skin injury in diabetics, the removal of hair may cause redness and bleeding from the follicle and skin injury, especially if the skin is thin and very sensitive. This may lead to an infection after waxing. Women with diabetes often will have very dry skins causing sensitivity and their pain threshold can be very low. Other indications for 'use with caution' when waxing, are people who have either high blood pressure, skin cancers, Parkinson's disease, multiple sclerosis, psoriasis, eczema, dementia, skin infections, eye disorders, or have suffered from a stroke. There can be many other contraindications when it comes to older people, especially for those who are in care. Because of the underlying problems they may have, waxing or tweezing should be done by a trained therapist.

The carer or relative and home user should not try any methods of hair removal on a person who is in care or very frail.

Facial hair disorders

Hirsutism This is an excess of hair growth in either male or female. In the female the hair growth may follow a male pattern and causes may be genetic, drug-induced, or hormonal. Hair can grow thickly on any part of the body and be more noticeable on parts of the face such as the chin, top lip or the forehead, growing more thickly on the sides, and down the sides of the face and neck. Women with this problem will also be prone to acne due to the over-production of sebum (oil).

Hair stubble These are short hairs left behind after waxing. They can be the result of new hair growth caused by shaving prior to waxing. They can be removed by tweezing.

Pseudo folliculitis This is a disorder of hair follicles. Hair follicles curve back into the skin causing several problems such as pustules, skin irritation, scarring and infections. Men are more prone to this disorder, especially those who have a darker skin.

Hair shaft defects This disorder is usually inherited. Conditions of the hair shaft cause the hairs to break and become brittle, beaded and abnormal in appearance.

The eyebrows

Eyebrows frame the face. The shape, length and thickness of the brows add definition to the eyes. The shape of the brows can change one's appearance. A person with very thin and high arched brows will give an impression of being surprised. A person who grows eyebrows which are thick, the hairs from both brows joining across the bridge of the nose, can give an angry impression. Properly shaped brows give definition and accentuate the eyes. Unfortunately, hair loss in the eyebrows can cause concern to many individuals. Hair loss can be the result of incorrect removal of hair, for example, over-tweezing, which may stunt re-growth or cause permanent hair loss. Other factors that can cause hair loss in the brows are certain medications such as chemotherapy, hormonal or endocrine conditions, skin diseases, thyroid disease, pregnancy and skin infections. As we age, the eyebrows lose colour and long grey and white strands of hair grow over the brow. In some older women, the hairs of the brow can disappear altogether, or they can grow in long coarse strands.[*] Not all women have problem eyebrows. Some women have beautifully shaped brows and are able to keep them maintained with ongoing beauty treatment.

---

[*]   The services of a beauty therapist are best used to remove unwanted eyebrow hair from a person in care.

Q. *What causes the hair on the brow to grow downwards?*

A. This could be genetic, or could be caused by improper removal of hair by waxing or tweezing. This problem can also be the result of a hormonal imbalance.

Q. *What causes the brow hair to grow so quickly?*

A. This problem could be due to a hormonal imbalance, thyroid problem, medication, or a nervous disorder. The brows will often need regular (fortnightly, to three-weekly) treatments to keep the shape maintained to its original form. Removing the hair without its bulb attached, or breaking the hair, will only lead to further problems as the hair will become coarser. In some cases there has been improvement for some of my clients who have this problem. However, while they still have an internal disorder, the problem will continue, but improvement is evident with beauty treatment.

Q. *What causes hairless patches in the brow?*

A. These may have been due to a skin infection that has damaged the follicle and hair shafts, inhibiting further re-growth. Other causes may be improper hair removal. Sometimes the patched area will still house fine translucent hair. If the patch has a few hairs, a colour tint may pick up on the translucent hair and give it colour.* This improves the eyebrow and gives the appearance of a natural eyebrow line. Some of my clients have found this method satisfactory.

Q. *How often should eyebrows be shaped?*

A. This depends on the individual. Generally treatments are given every four to six weeks or less, which is much the same for waxing.

Q. *What is the correct shape for an eyebrow?*

A. The hair should follow the brow line above the eye socket. To measure how the brow line should be shaped, the following instructions may help.

---

*   Never use a colour tint on an eyebrow if there is any skin disorder, infection, or if the person is sensitive to peroxide which is mixed in with the colour tint.

1   Hold an eyebrow pencil to the side of the nose. The pencil should line up with the inner edge of the brow (where the hair is thickest) and should start above the nose where the top of the nose meets with the eyebrow. Draw a soft line at the brow edge.

2   Hold the pencil from the side of the nostril and hold diagonally from the nostril side to the outside edge of the eye where it meets the brow line. Draw another line. This will be the correct length.

3   To find the right position for the 'arch' in the brow, hold the pencil parallel to the outside edge of the iris (or, for smaller eyes, it may need to come more towards the middle of the iris). This is the highest part of the arch. Draw a line. Now there are three lines. Connect them and this will give an idea of how the brow will look. Unwanted hair growing outside the line is then removed.

Having eyebrows professionally shaped for the first time is money well spent. This saves a lot of time, and alleviates first-time disasters. Once the brows have been treated, you will have a better idea of how the brows should look with their new shape.

Steps to shaping the eyebrows

Step one   Clean the area with an antiseptic lotion and remove any makeup.

Step two   Work out the shape of the eyebrow as described above and apply a small dot of aloe gel to help minimize stings.

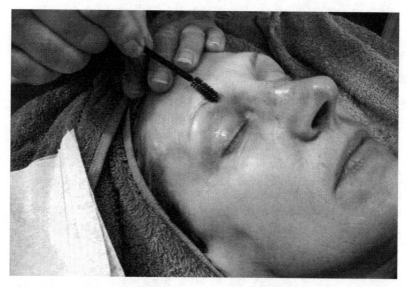

Plate 4.1 Before having a facial, the client has her eyebrows shaped. The therapist is using a mascara wand as an alternative to an eyebrow brush.

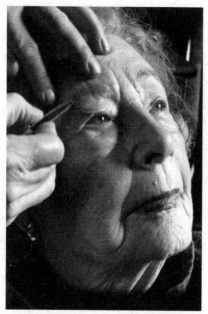

Plate 4.2 The therapist visits a client in a nursing home. The client is seated in a chair while her eyebrows are being shaped.

Step three   Using a brow comb or a clean disposable mascara wand, brush hair upwards and outwards; comb down the unwanted hair strands that are to be removed.

Step four   With the opposite hand pull and hold the skin tight at the edge of the eyebrow where it thins. Holding the tweezers in the other hand, start to pull out unwanted hairs one at a time, pulling in the direction of the growth of the hair.

Step five   Once the hairs have been removed, clean the area and hold a cold calendula compress to help minimize any redness.

Be careful when removing the hair from the follicle. If you break the hair from its bulb you will leave stubble (bulb and part of hair) in the follicle and it will grow back more coarsely.

Useful websites

The websites listed below are current at the time of my research on 30 June 2008 before publication.

Brow Makeover Makeup Tips (2008)
www.eyebrows.com

Ingrown Hair Solutions (2008)
www.ingrown-hair-solutions.com

Glossary

Aesthetician	A person who is artistic in the application of beauty treatments and skilled in the removal of unwanted hair. Another title for Beauty Therapist or Beautician.
Coarse	Refers to strong terminal hair.

Erythema   Redness of the skin caused by conges-
tion of the capillaries in the lower layers of the skin. It occurs with any skin
injury, infection or inflammation.

Follicle   A sac or pouch-like depression or cavity.

Hair bulb   The bulbous expansion at the lower
end of the hair root.

Hair follicle   A pouch-like depression in the skin in
which the hair develops from the ma-
trix at its base and grows to emerge
from its opening on the body surface.

Hair shaft   Structure of the hair which is seen
above the scalp. It is divided into three
layers: 1 The cuticle – the outermost
layer made up of dead skin cells which
protects the inner layers of the hair. 2
The cortex, or middle layer which is
the largest portion of the hair made up
of melanin. 3 The medulla which is
the innermost layer.

Hairstrand   A threadlike structure, especially the
specialized epidermal structures devel-
oping from a papilla sunk in the
corium.

Hormonal   Hormones act as chemical messengers
to body organs stimulating certain life
processes and retarding others as in
growth, reproduction and control of
metabolic processes.

Keratin   A protein that is the principal constituent of the epidermis, hair, nails, horny
tissues and the organic matrix of the
enamel in teeth.

Melanin   A dark, sulphur-containing pigment
normally found in the hair, the skin,

ciliary body, choroid of the eye, pigment layer of the retina and certain nerve cells. It occurs abnormally in certain tumours, known as melanomas, and is sometimes excreted in the urine, when such tumours are present (melanuria).

Melanocytes
Any of the dendritic clear cells of the epidermis that synthesize tyrosinase and, within their melanosomes, the pigment melanin. The melanosomes are then transferred from melanocytes to keratinocytes.

Papule
Blind pimple containing no fluid which varies in size.

Pustule
Pimple containing pus, appearing at the mouth of the follicle, a red area with a central core of pus.

Tweezing
The use of small pincers for taking up small objects or removing unwanted hair from the body.

Wax
A sticky substance made with gum resin or honey and used to remove unwanted hair from parts of the body.

CHAPTER 5

Nutrition and Health

Nutrition is a complex topic that I am unable to discuss fully in this chapter. My aim is to give the reader an understanding of the importance of nutrition and the role it plays to maintain a healthy body including the health of our skin, nails and hair.

Nutrition

Nutrition is the relationship between foods and the health of the human body. Evidence of good nutrition is revealed by signs of healthy hair, fingernails and especially the skin. As the old saying goes 'what goes in, shows through the skin'. Good nutrition is essential to the body for its normal development and functioning. Normal reproduction, growth, maintenance, optimum activity levels, resistance to infection and bodily repair all depend on this. Proper nutrition means that all the essential nutrients, carbohydrates, fats, protein, vitamins, minerals and water, are supplied and utilized in an adequate balance to maintain optimal health and well-being. Nutritional deficiencies may result in disease whenever adequate amounts of these essential nutrients are not provided to the tissues that must function for long periods of time. Poor nutrition is evident when a person begins to feel sluggish, tired, breathless, stressed and ill. All of the above can be due to lack of certain vitamins and minerals in the diet. Other signs are: dull splitting hair, nail disorders and skin problems. Dehydration of the skin is another sign of nutritional deficiency. Some other problems that relate to a poor diet are as follows.

Faddish foods Weight gain caused by eating fatty and sugar laden foods leads to poor health. In some people, there are certain fats that will increase free radical activity within the body to accelerate ageing. This is a common problem among many individuals who rely on 'fast foods' due to their hectic and stressed lifestyles.

Smoking Smoking can double the rate of premature facial wrinkling. It also discolours the skin, giving a leathery texture when a person continues to smoke for a long period of time. Other smoking related problems are skin and nail disorders, hair nutrient deficiencies, dehydration and other internal disorders. Smoking also causes bad breath and an unpleasant body odour.

Stress The body quickly loses its reserves of vitamins when under pressure, especially vitamins B and C, and the mineral zinc. Good nutrition is an effective way to deal with stress. A daily intake of green vegetables, fresh fruit, whole grain cereals, nuts, seeds and dried fruit will help boost the immune system.

Exercise Poor nutrition and a sedentary lifestyle will slow down the flow of lymph in the body, causing a build-up of toxins. Lack of activity affects the digestive process which may lead to constipation and other internal disorders. Regular exercise will boost the circulatory system, help eliminate body wastes, tone body muscles, reduce weight, increase body energy, and maintain good health and well-being. Exercising over a period of time will help improve the skin, nails and hair condition, when good nutrition is combined with the exercise.

Vitamins and minerals

Vitamins and minerals are essential for good health and optimally should be obtained through natural foods. Deficiencies are still a problem in certain parts of the world, especially third-world countries where population growth is higher and food sources are minimal. In developed countries where a variety of food is plentiful, nutritional deficiencies should not be a problem. Unfortunately, a large percentage of people are on the borderline of health safety, mainly due to the fact that they have a poorly balanced diet. A less active lifestyle could mean less desire for food, making it more difficult to obtain all the necessary nutrients. Those who consume large amounts of sugary foods, saturated fats, alcohol, all of which supply very little vitamins or minerals, are risking poor nutrition.

Quality of food is important and whole fresh natural foods are the best. In developed countries, the quality of food can vary, and many food products decrease in nutrient value due to the way they are grown and processed. For commercial production, plants are grown on soil that has been treated with fertilizers and chemical sprays which deplete vitamin and mineral efficiency. The water used to irrigate the plants is sometimes treated with chemicals. Plants are often grown on a minimal amount of soil thereby depleting their ability to obtain full nutrient value, thus creating an inferior food, deficient in vitamins and other food components.

A few decades ago, food was mainly eaten 'in season' and many people grew their own food, thereby retaining its vitamin and mineral effectiveness. Today food is preserved and stored so that we can eat foods that are generally 'out of season' throughout much of the year. Preservation and irradiation* methods are used to allow us this choice. Unseasonal food, forced to ripen and placed on the market shelf, may have less than its full vitamin and mineral value and this is one reason why vitamin supplements have become popular recently.

Organically grown food is a better option. The plants are grown on soil that is fertilized with natural organic material (house scraps, animal manure, garden waste, etc.) and no synthetic chemicals are used. The plants have plenty of room to grow and therefore have the ability to absorb all the nutrients they require. Organically grown food is generally harvested in season and the taste, quality and smell are excellent. The colour of organically grown food is its own natural colour. Therefore it does not show a bright vivid colour with a shiny surface as do its synthetically enhanced cousins, produced 'out of season', and coated in a preservative, to maintain a longer shelf life.

Shelf life for organically grown food is short and the food will discolour quickly, as no preservatives or synthetic colours have been added. In all foods, vitamins and minerals begin to decrease once food has been:

1   exposed to the elements

2   cut or sliced

3   over-cooked

---

*   The food irradiation process involves food being placed in a chamber and exposed to gamma radiation from a radioactive source. The rays kill insects, bacteria and viruses, preventing some fresh fruit and vegetables from ripening quickly and thereby extending their shelf life.

4   allowed to wilt and age

5   allowed to go rancid.

Nutrition for older people

As we age, our calorie requirements lessen, but we need the same amount of nutrients as before. In older people nutrient absorption declines, reducing the levels of zinc and vitamins B6 and D, affecting the body's immunity and general health. The decrease in calorie needs is due to slower metabolism and, in most people, lessened activity. Medication can increase the risks of poor nutrition owing to the effects of drug-nutrient interactions. Vitamins affected by drug interaction are the B group, and vitamins K, D, A and C.

The importance of vitamin D

Vitamin D is involved in the absorption of calcium and in metabolism. Recently vitamin D has been found to have a much larger role in supporting the immune system and in regulating brain chemistry to ward off depression. Too much covering up and avoiding the sun may have done more harm than good. However, we need to have a balance. Exposure of the skin to the sun should never involve burning.

> In recent times, many Australian aged-care facilities tend to encourage staff and residents to spend time in the sun daily to obtain adequate vitamin D. Of course some people have very sensitive skin, and may need to have vitamin D supplements, but the free resource from the sun is probably better and more therapeutic.

Nutrition impairment

Among older people, multiple illnesses and disabilities are common. Diseases cause impairments at the organ and cellular level, resulting in disability and loss of personal functions required for everyday independent living (e.g. eating). Common conditions with nutritional implications in older people are:

1 arteriosclerosis

2 arthritis

3 hypertension

4 heart disease

5 orthopaedic impairments

6 chronic sinusitis

7 diabetes mellitus

8 cataracts

9 deafness and hearing loss

10 haemorrhoids

11 blindness

12 constipation.

Other factors that lead to poor nutrition are recent hospitalization, surgery, trauma, infection, or required assistance in feeding. Nutritional deficiency can affect older people who suffer some types of dementia. Low body mass is quite common in demented frail people, taking into account any other illness they may be suffering. Depressive disorders are common among older people who reside in nursing homes or other aged-care facilities. Older people living alone can suffer from weight loss, lack of appetite and poor nutrition because of the inability to shop, prepare food, and feed themselves due to their disability, impairments in taste and smell, oral medications, depression, lack of appetite and (in some agitated persons) increased energy needs.

Factors that may lead to a person's lack of interest in eating are:

1   religious beliefs, as certain foods may be forbidden in their diet

2   foods that upset the digestive system

3   the inability to eat at certain times

4   unappetizing food

5   food too cold or hot

6   foods that are unpalatable

7   stress, both emotional and physical

8   depression

9   other rational or irrational personal beliefs.

Dentures and gum problems

Nutritional impairment can also be the result of poor fitting dentures, sore gums and mouth. Many older persons have lost most of their teeth and have difficulty in chewing. Some have lost all their teeth and wear both top and bottom denture plates. Gum shrinkage is common. It can cause improper fitting of dentures which can lead to soreness in the gums and gum ulcers. In some cases, this is known as 'the hidden pain', as there are frail older people who are unable to communicate and will suffer in silence, unbeknown to the carer. Some indications that an older frail person may be having problems with their dentures or gums are:

1   dribbling

2   sucking on fingers and dribbling

3   sensitivity to being touched in and around the mouth

4   movement of dentures in the mouth, causing pain

5   swelling in the gums and mouth

6   bad breath (this can also result from medication and illness).

Should any of these signs be evident, the carer or relative should take the person to their dentist or have the dentures fitted properly by an orthodontist. Seek medical attention for any infection.

Intake of water

As a main constituent of body fluids and as the universal solvent, water acts as a medium in which substances are transported to and from the cells. Water nourishes the body internally and externally. Elimination of wastes depends on water. Water is vital for life. About 75 per cent of your body and almost all of your blood is made up of water. A person can survive a month or more without food, but without water the survival rate is much shorter, especially in hot climates. If you lose 20 per cent of the water in your body, you could die of dehydration. In a temperate climate the body needs about 3 litres of water a day. If a dry diet is consumed, then the water intake needs to be greater. A diet containing plenty of fresh fruit and vegetables would require less water as both provide 60–90 per cent of our water intake.

The importance of perspiration

Sweat glands are connected to blood capillaries in the dermis (true skin) and produce liquid containing water, salts and waste materials known as sweat. To eliminate body wastes and control body temperature, sweat travels to the surface of the skin in ducts through the pores. When you use more body energy, you will sweat more and the body will heat up, therefore increasing the volume of sweat in an effort to cool the body down. Your body will let you know if you have lost a lot of water by sweating and you will feel thirsty.

It is important to wash yourself regularly, especially if you sweat a lot. Sweat does not smell, but it may, if bacteria are involved. Main culprits for sweat odour are: spicy foods, garlic, smoking, alcohol consumption, medication, illness and hygiene neglect.

Water for life

When you feel thirsty, an alarm signal sent by the brain will tell you that you need to drink. If your body does not contain enough fluid, less urine will be produced. You need to drink to maintain hydration for all bodily functions including the function of the kidneys. Fluid intake is vital for your body. If you expel more fluid than you take in, this could result in serious health problems.

The colour of your urine may indicate if you are not taking in enough fluid and some of the signs are:

1   the passing of yellow straw-coloured urine throughout the day

2   frequent passing of urine in small quantities

3   very little output of urine throughout the day.

If you are having the required intake of daily fluids and the above signs are evident, this may indicate that an internal imbalance is the cause.

A healthy sign of fluid intake is that the quantity of urine passed through the day will often be of a light to clear colour. The colour of urine can change if certain foods with a strong dye have been eaten, such as beetroot.

Medication, vitamin supplements, hormonal changes during pregnancy or menopause and illness may also cause a change in the colour of urine. Other signs which may appear are pain, discomfort, cloudy urine, a strong ammoniacal or sweet sickly odour, infection and incontinence. If there are signs of an abnormality, a medical practitioner should be consulted.

Water intake for older people

Water requirements are particularly important for older people. Thirst mechanisms are weak, levels of body water are low, and the ability to concentrate urine decreases. Many older people are on diuretics which cause increased excretion of water. Some older people will favour their daily intake of coffee, tea or sweet drinks in place of their daily water requirement. This can contribute to dehydration and constipation, leading to many discomforts and illness. Taking into consideration all the facts that cause nutritional impairment, it is often difficult to educate some older persons as to the benefits of a good diet. For the carer, or relative of a person in their care, it can be very distressing and be seen as a 'no win' situation. (It is like taking a horse to water, but being unable to get it to drink.) Helping to maintain a healthy diet in an older frail person experiencing illness, chronic pain, disabilities and taking regular medication, is one of the most difficult tasks for any health practitioner or carer.

Useful websites

The websites listed below are current at the time of my research on 30 June 2008 before publication.

Felton Grimwade and Brickford Pty Ltd (2004) Elderly Nutrition.
www.fgb.com.au/NaturalUses/ElderlyNutrition.htm

Food Nutrition Australia (2006)
www.foodnut.com.au

British Nutrition Foundation
www.nutrition.org.uk

Glossary

Angina pectoris   Signs are a deep aching, crushing pain in the chest radiating perhaps to the left arm, or up into the neck and jaw.

Affects mainly men in their 40s and over, whose arteries have been seriously narrowed by atherosclerosis.

Arteriosclerosis Hardening of the arteries. Usually occurs in the elderly and those who have a high blood level of cholesterol.

Arthritis Inflammation of a joint.

Atherosclerosis A form of arteriosclerosis. A condition underlying the current epidemic of coronary thrombosis (heart disease) and stroke.

Cataracts Opacity in the lens of the eye causing defective vision.

Cell The basic structural unit of living organisms.

Constipation Inability to have a bowel movement, stools become hard and dry and are difficult to pass. Inactive people, people on low fibre diets, and those taking some medications may suffer from constipation.

Coronary heart disease The left and right coronary arteries divide into smaller arteries that supply blood to the heart. Narrowing or blockage of the coronary arteries gives rise to angina or a heart attack.

Cortisone An anti-inflammatory agent, for adrenal replacement therapy.

Deficiency The shortage of an essential nutrient in the diet.

Dementia Loss of mental capacity.

Diabetes mellitus A syndrome in which the basic defect is absence or a shortage of the pancreatic hormone insulin. Maturity onset diabetes has a slower onset, in middle

	age or later years, and can usually be controlled by diet alone or with special tablets.
Gamma radiation	Electromagnetic radiation of shorter wavelength than x-rays.
Haemorrhoids	Commonly called 'piles'. Veins around the anus are abnormally dilated. They can be very painful and sometimes the tiny vessels will erupt, causing bleeding during a bowel motion.
Hypertension	High blood pressure.
Metabolism	The natural building and breakdown of substances by the cells of the body.
Nutrition	By which the body uses food for energy, maintenance and growth. Vitamins, minerals, carbohydrates, protein, fats (omega 3 and omega 6 – unsaturated fats) are the essential nutrients required daily to maintain a healthy body.
Obesity	Excessive accumulation of fat in the body; increase in weight beyond that considered desirable with regard to age, height and bone structure.
Orthodontist	A dentist who specializes in the correction of irregularities of the teeth and jaws.
Orthopaedics	Branch of medicine dealing with the correction of diseased, deformed or injured bones or muscles.
Osteoarthritis	A degenerative disease of the joints, usually accompanied by pain and stiffness.
Osteoporosis	A bone condition in which calcium, the basic content of bone, drops to a dangerously low level. The bones

soften and may bend, break or col-
lapse. This is common among women
and affects those in their 50s and
above.

Rheumatoid arthritis (medication)   A chronic systemic disease with inflammatory changes occurring
throughout the body's connective tissues.

Stroke   A blockage of a blood vessel in the
brain depriving parts of the brain of a
blood supply, resulting in loss of con-
sciousness, paralysis, or other symptoms depending on the site and extent
of brain damage.

The Skin

In this chapter where I give reference to cosmetic use and medical treatment for skin problems and disorders, I cannot recommend drug or cosmetic brands for skin disorders or skin blemishes, as each person is different. Assessment by a medical person may be needed for advice on medicated creams or by a beauty therapist for cosmetic lotions and creams. It is known that some natural therapies may help to soothe and minimize inflammatory problems in skin disorders. I mention a few of these therapies and it is for the consumer to choose the therapy which will most benefit them. Persons under medical care must seek advice from their medical practitioner before incorporating any natural therapy with their treatment.

The skin

The skin is the most important sensory organ, and renews itself most rapidly. Its function is to help regulate body temperature, protect the body, eliminate wastes, and synthesize vitamin D and it also responds to certain stimuli: temperature, pressure and pain.

The skin is the first line of defence in its protection of internal organs from the external world. It also has its own immune system protecting it against foreign bodies such as irritants, viruses, bacteria, parasites and fungi.

The structure of the skin

There are two main layers of the skin.

The first layer is called the epidermis, the outermost layer which protects the body with its sheath of drying and dead cells. The epidermis consists of 15 to 25 layers of closely connected cells. These vary in thickness in different parts of the body according to its functional need. The epidermis is thicker on the soles of our feet and palms of our hands, thinner in the area of our eyes and eyelids. Melanocytes are present in the epidermis and these are the cells which produce the pigment melanin, giving colour to our skin and hair. When these cells stop producing melanin, hair begins to turn grey, and, eventually, white. The skin will become pale pink to white leaving patches on any part of the body that is affected by the decrease or absence of melanocytes.

The second layer is called the dermis, the inner layer of the skin and it is also referred to as the 'true skin'. The dermis consists of sweat glands, hair follicles, hair bulbs, blood and lymphatic vessels, oil glands, nerves, connective tissue such as collagen, and elastic fibres.

Below these two layers is the hypodermis. It is made of subcutaneous fat which protects the body and helps maintain heat. This layer lies between the skin and the muscles and bones of our body. With age and sun damage, loss of elasticity in the fibres of the skin will cause wrinkling. There are more elastic fibres in the face and neck area, hence wrinkling is more prominent here.

The skin through the decades

The ageing process

There are two processes in skin ageing.

1   **Natural ageing**, also called intrinsic, or inherent ageing. This is our natural biological ageing which is determined by our genes.

2   **The environment and ageing** also called extrinsic ageing, because it is outside the body. The environment plays an important role in this ageing process. Exposure to the elements, such as UV rays, chemical pollutants and mechanical influences such as heat or cold increase the ageing process. Lifestyle influences, such as smoking, alcohol consumption, drugs, disturbed sleep, stress, nervous habitual facial expressions, skin care neglect, nutrition impairment and hygiene neglect also accelerate the ageing process.

As the body ages through the decades, the skin goes through a few changes.

The 20s

In line with the natural biological ageing process, the skin should look its best at this age. Cell turnover is at its peak and the skin complexion should be in good condition after undergoing the major changes of adolescence.

Cosmetically

This is the time to start taking good care of your skin, incorporating a skin care routine with daily cleansing and moisturizing. Sunscreen protection should be worn and skin should not be overexposed to UV rays.

Unfortunately there are many individuals in this age group who still suffer acne and have oily skin problems, especially males. Excess oiliness and pimples are often the result of ongoing hormonal adjustment. Cosmetically, foaming cleansers and cosmetic soap bars may be suitable, but for severe acne it is advisable to seek medical advice.

The 30s

Cell turnover and sebum (oil) production decreases in this decade. Fine lines around the eyes and lips begin to appear, more so if there is lifestyle abuse. Pigmentation such as freckles and other spots may start to show as a result of sun exposure. Other brown marks such as chloasma can appear around the eyes or face, especially during pregnancy or whilst taking the contraceptive pill, from sun exposure or as a factor of heredity. Acne and oiliness can still be a problem in the T-zone area.

Cosmetically

Exfoliate the skin two to three times weekly, daily cleanse and moisturize. A weekly face mask or steam treatment may be of benefit. An eye cream or gel applied at night will help soothe and moisturize fine lines around the eye area. You may also find that the skin care products you have used since your 20s are no longer suitable. Visit a beauty therapist to have an up-dated skin analysis.

The 40s

At this age, the protective film (or skin barrier) on the skin's surface becomes less effective in the retention of moisture. This leads to a higher percentage of moisture loss, causing dehydration and thinning of the skin, making it less efficient in its protective capacity. Fine lines, broken veins, wrinkles and a few 'age spots' become more obvious. Daily cleansing and moisturizing skin care treatment is a must.

Cosmetically

The skin will require cleansing and moisturizing twice daily. Twice weekly exfoliate the skin and apply a mask treatment once a week. A regular facial treatment with your beauty therapist will help improve the skin texture of your face and neck.

The 50s

The change in the skin during this decade is the result of our lifestyle plus the effects of our natural biological ageing process. Some individuals will look healthy and younger while others will look much older suffering many skin ailments. No matter how well we have looked after our skin, changes will occur governed by our natural biological clock. In this decade, the production of sebum (oil) slows and the outer layer of the skin loses resilience, while the renewal of cell turnover is less than 60 per cent. After menopause the production of oestrogen, the skin's 'youth' hormone, slows down and the skin becomes much drier. Lack of oestrogen thins the skin and reduces the strength of collagen, the skin's structural support system. Broken capillaries, skin cysts, spots, rosacea, moles, warts, other skin problems may appear. Lines around the eyes and wrinkles can become more noticeable.

Cosmetically
The use of a rich moisture cream twice daily, regular exfoliation and mask treatment with herbal infusions may benefit the skin. Regular facial treatments with a beauty therapist would benefit circulation, lymphatic flow and stimulation of the skin's natural moisturizing agent, keeping it soft, smooth and hydrated.

The 60s onwards

As the ageing process continues into the 60s and beyond, certain changes in the skin are easily visible. The skin becomes more dehydrated and dries out. It becomes thinner, and then it is vulnerable to the elements which can be the cause of many skin problems. Loss of elastic fibres in the dermis and decreasing resilience will cause the skin to become loose and wrinkled. Many spots, skin growths and marks appear on some individuals. The cells in the tissues regenerate more slowly, cell repair slows, and poor circulation also causes slower healing and skin repair. Not all older persons will have wrinkles or skin complaints, as this may be due to their genetic makeup and an earlier healthy active lifestyle.

Cosmetically

Most mature skins would benefit from night creams or a rich moisturizing cream. Gentle cleansing and face massage would help stimulate circulation and the skin's natural moisturizing agent. Mask treatments would benefit mature skins.

Skin problems

There are many skin problems and disorders that require the expertise of a medical practitioner such as a dermatologist for diagnosis and treatment. The questions I shall endeavour to answer about skin problems are the ones with which I am familiar in my work and most asked about by many clients. The home user and carer will be familiar with some skin complaints, but may not know how to address them. In older people and the medically frail, there are individuals who have a number of skin problems and skin disorders which may need medical attention, therefore it is best to get advice before using a cosmetic cream or any natural products for skin care for treatment.

The questions asked by clients mostly relate to acne, age spots, allergies, birth marks, blackheads, broken capillaries, bruising, cherry angiomas, chloasma, cold sores, dermatitis (includes allergies), eczema, erythema, freckles, moles, pimples, psoriasis, rosacea, rashes, seborrheic keratosis, skin cancers, skin tags, warts, whiteheads, varicose veins and vitiligo.

Acne

Q. What causes acne?

A. Acne occurs if the hair follicles become blocked and the normal bacteria of the skin multiply within the clogged pores. The most common blemishes which occur are blackheads, whiteheads, pimples, blind pimples, cysts and scars. The four main influences of this process are hormones, diet, medication and certain products used on the skin. In teenage years, the skin produces so many secretions that the ducts cannot eliminate them, causing retention, blockage and infection.

Cosmetically

For mild acne, use a cleanser suitable for acne or a cosmetic soap bar. A lavender infusion used as a toner or steam treatment can be incorporated into the skin care routine. For pustules that have become infected, the use of an antiseptic or antibacterial cleanser would be suitable. There are various forms of acne and those who suffer with several break-outs may need a medicated cleanser and a topical cream. Cosmetics only aid in cleansing and moisturizing and some products may minimize mild acne but they do not cure it.

Medically

Acne is a skin disease. It needs medical attention especially in severe cases.

Alternatives

Herbal medicine, nutrition, acupuncture, acupressure may benefit mild cases.

Q. What causes acne rosacea?

A. This is caused by deterioration of the skin, particularly through sun exposure, causing infection in the hair follicles and skin glands. People with naturally dry skin are more prone to this condition. In effect, the skin barrier has broken down. Other agents which may increase the severity of rosacea are alcohol, bad nutrition, smoking and diminished hormonal activity, consistent with ageing. Rosacea is a chronic inflammatory skin disorder which appears as a butterfly shape on the face, including the cheeks and nose. It can also include the forehead and chin in severe cases. Rosacea affects men and women from their 30s but is more common in post-menopausal women. The pink colour which forms is due to the increased blood flow created as a result of the infection.

Cosmetically
Light cleansing and a moisturizer with SPF 30+ would be suitable for sensitive skin or those exhibiting a mild form of rosacea.

Medically
People with severe rosacea need medical attention and possibly antibiotics.

Alternatives
These may include aromatherapy, face reflexology or flower remedies.

Brown spots

Q. *What are the large brown spots that appear on older people's hands?*

A. Actinic lentigo, also called age spots or 'liver spots' are more noticeable on middle-aged to an older persons but bear no relation to the liver. These brown spots are similar to freckles being yellow to brownish in colour and slightly raised. They appear on sun-exposed areas of the body and are purely related to ageing. The spots commonly appear on the back of the hands, lower arms and face, and are not pre-cancerous.

Cosmetically

Skin care application does not affect these spots. A usual skin care routine, plus a tinted moisture cream with an SPF 30+ would be suitable.

Medically

Cryotherapy treatment where liquid nitrogen is applied by a cotton wool bud or spray gun to the affected area kills the superficial cells. A brown patch will appear and after ten days it will dry and fall off, leaving the skin clear. This treatment is performed by a medical practitioner such as a dermatologist. If exposed to sunlight after the treatment, the UV rays may cause ulceration and blistering, especially in older people.

Other brown spots that appear on the face and other parts of the body which have been affected by sunlight are commonly freckles or ephelides. Freckles are small, flat, light-brown macules which darken on exposure to the sun. They have a higher incidence in fair-skinned individuals and especially women with red hair.

Cosmetically

Normal skin care routine is carried out. Use a tinted moisture cream with an SPF 30+ or a sun protection cream. In a beauty salon, the therapist may have a product that can help reduce the intensity of the colour in the spot or mark.

Medically

Topical bleaching creams and peeling pastes can be purchased through a pharmacist. If the spots or marks are exposed to sunlight again, they will re-appear.

Allergies

Q. *Why do some people suffer more with allergy problems than others?*

A. Allergies can occur as a result of exposure to certain chemicals, pollutants or plants, or consumption of certain food products and medications. However, the symptoms may only manifest themselves later in life. Histamine is the primary chemical that initiates the symptoms of an allergy. The immune system produces large amounts of antibodies that cause special mast cells to release powerful chemicals into the bloodstream in an attempt to destroy the harmful invaders. Some people are prone to suffer with allergy problems most of their lives especially if they have been exposed to allergens during childhood. Generally, a person does not develop the symptoms of an allergy the first time they come into contact with an allergen. It takes continued or repeated exposure before symptoms develop. An inflammatory response is triggered once the immune system considers the substance harmful. This is why suddenly you may start to react to a certain product such as detergents, cosmetics or jewellery that you have been using or wearing for a long time.

Q. *What are the most common signs of skin allergies?*

A. Skin allergies can range from mild to major. The skin may show redness, swelling (oedema), a rash, dryness where dead skin cells accumulate on the skin surface, dandruff, blistering or weals. The main culprits can be cosmetics, detergents, plant materials, jewellery, chemicals, medication, food products or dander in animal fur. The following are some common skin allergies:

Urticaria – Hives or nettle rash

This skin condition usually shows up as a rash of itchy, raised, localized swellings, called weals. Weals are white blister-like lumps and are the result of fluid leaking out through dilated blood vessels. Weals are common with most allergic reactions. (Scratching, thus making the skin bleed, can worsen the problem, as open skin lesions are prone to infection.)

Rashes

Rash can be a term used to describe almost any skin condition. Erythema (redness) in the affected area is the most common manifestation. A rash appears when the skin has come into contact with a substance that has caused an allergic reaction. Other conditions may accompany the rash, such as weals, swellings and bumps. Rashes consisting of spots, dryness, itching or inflammation are common in a number of skin conditions. A rash that develops with a raised temperature is more likely to be an infection and a rash with a fever should be treated by a medical practitioner.

Q. *What are the most common forms of dermatitis?*

A. Dermatitis is an inflammatory process in the skin. It can be caused by infection, physical trauma, chemicals and allergies.

Contact Dermatitis

Contact dermatitis is caused by direct contact with a substance either by ingestion, inhalation or direct contact usually on the skin. Once you have developed an allergy to a certain material or substance, the reaction will continue with ongoing contact or recur with renewed contact. Contact dermatitis often affects the hands and arms, though it can appear in other parts of the body. The skin can become very dry, itchy and flaky. In severe cases, there can be painful cracking of the dried skin and blistering. Common culprits are detergents, soaps, jewellery, zips, watches, bra hooks, coins, scissors, cosmetics, nail varnish, newsprint, rubber, leather, chemicals, hair colours or dyes and dander in animal fur and bird feathers.

Cosmetically
You may use an emollient cream and moisture cream specifically for dried and cracking skin to protect it from water and harsh weather conditions.

Medically

You may need a topical medicated cream that can be used with a cosmetic cream, but for a severe dermatitis disorder you will need to seek medical attention.

Alternatives

These may include aromatherapy, flower remedies, acupuncture and face reflexology.

Atopic Eczema

This is a form of dermatitis, a systemic allergy due to ingestion or inhalation of a substance. The most common of these allergies is to cow's milk or other dairy products. This type of dermatitis affects babies and young children. Atopic eczema occurs without any obvious surface contact with an irritating substance. Adults can be affected, especially if they were prone to this condition in childhood, or if it runs in the family. Sufferers of atopic eczema are more likely to be prone to other allergic conditions such as hay fever, asthma, etc. The symptoms can range from a mild episode of redness and itching to chronic dry, scaly, red, itchy and weeping sores. Treatment cannot always cure the condition but a number of remedies are available to ease the discomfort.

Cosmetically

Use an emollient and moisture cream for sensitive skin. Some new cosmetic creams may contain ingredients to soothe skin irritation and help discomfort. A cosmetic cream in some cases may be used with a topical medicated cream.

Medically

Severe cases of atopic eczema should be treated by a medical practitioner.

Alternatives

These may include aromatherapy, reflexology, Bowen massage, herbal medicine. Avocado, calendula and primrose oil may be good alternatives to soothe irritation.

Seborrheic dermatitis (SD) (or seborrheic eczema)

This is another common skin condition that can range from mild to severe. It is a chronic inflammatory condition that mainly affects the scalp and face. It can begin at almost any age but usually affects adults in their twenties and thirties. It also can become worse in older people and affects men more frequently than women. It causes flaking, redness and irritation on many parts of the body especially in areas of hair growth and the scalp. SD often starts on the scalp as a mild case of dandruff and usually does not get any worse. In some cases, it can worsen by spreading to other parts of the body, especially the face and neck. The eyebrows may be affected and will have small clumps of yellow plaques among the hair growth and along the bridge of the nose between the eyebrows. The skin can appear shiny, red and inflamed becoming infected and damaged. Agents that can cause SD to appear are shampoos, colour dyes, cosmetics and soaps. Other conditions that can make this problem worse are exposure to strong sunlight and stress.

Cosmetically

Use skin creams designed for hypersensitive skins and use a medicated shampoo designed for clearing dandruff. There are also shampoos with natural herbal ingredients influential in combating dandruff and these can be very helpful.

Medically

From the pharmacy, anti-yeast or antifungal creams may be helpful for other areas of the body. For severe cases, a medical practitioner or dermatologist may prescribe a steroid cream or ointment.

Alternatives

Avocado oil rubbed over the skin may help soothe inflammation. Primrose oil and some herbal remedies have been known to help individuals with mild cases.

Q. *Why does sun exposure cause a rash when taking certain medications?*

A. Certain antibiotics, anti-inflammatory drugs and diuretics can cause a condition known as photosensitivity. Photosensitivity refers to the skin's increased sensitivity to the sun. Other causes of photosensitivity are a direct result of exposure, chemicals in sunscreens, perfumes and some cosmetics. Once you stop using the offending products and stop taking any medication, the condition will possibly disappear.

Do not stop using or taking any medication unless advised by your medical practitioner.

Q. *What causes prickly heat? (Sweat or heat rash)*

A. Prickly heat produces a rash that develops when the sweat ducts become swollen and blocked. It occurs mainly on people in warmer climates and is associated with excessive sweating. Sweat ducts become blocked when the temperature rises and small blood vessels under the skin widen. The skin becomes congested as the tissues swell, blocking the pores of the skin preventing the escape of perspiration. Prickly heat tends to affect the body in areas where sweat accumulates such as the chest, armpits, elbows, waist, or groin.

Overweight people may find that they suffer from this condition frequently on hot days. People who are overweight have less ability to cope with heat but it can affect people of any size.

Moles

Q. *What causes moles to form and do they need to be checked regularly?*

A. It is not known for sure why moles develop. However, it is known that sun exposure in early life initiates this process. There is also a hereditary tendency. Moles comprise pigment-producing cells, called melanocytes. They may be various shades of brown, and some are skin coloured. From middle age, any moles that remain are often light pink or colourless, lumpy and raised. They can appear on any part of the body and become raised over a period of time. Some can become very large and hair may grow out of them. Moles are harmless until they begin to change or become a nuisance when clothing catches on them which will cause bleeding or discomfort.

Medically

Moles can be removed by a medical practitioner such as a dermatologist.

Q. *What are these hard brown marks on the forehead and neck?*

A. These marks are called Seborrhoeic warts (Seborrhoeic keratosis). They are rough warts and can look like moles. They are harmless growths that are slightly raised and feel rough and dry. They can range from small to large patches and show a light brown to black colour. They can become very itchy and annoying when clothing rubs over the surface of the wart. SK can be found on most parts of the body; however they appear more in the forehead near the temples, under the bust line, sides of the face, and backs of the hands, especially in older people.

Cosmetically

Cosmetics can be used to cover warts. Do not try to pull or pick at the warts, as they can bleed and may cause an infection.

---

* Older people who develop new moles should have them checked. Any mole that starts to change in size, colour or shape, or begins to bleed or weep fluids, must be checked by a medical practitioner.

Medically
They can be removed. Unfortunately they have a tendency to regrow.

Q. *How can you tell if a mole has turned into a skin cancer?*

A. If a mole or spot (for example, a freckle) shows any change, and you become aware that something is different, do not hesitate to have it checked by a medical practitioner. The following explanations of skin cancer will not make any recommendations for cosmetic use or alternative therapies, as these conditions must be seen by a medical practitioner.

Malignant melanoma (MM)

Melanoma can develop in normal skin and in pre-existing moles. It can appear anywhere on the body and even in areas that have not been affected by the sun. This disease can affect people of all ages, post-adolescence. The form of treatment for MM will depend on whether it has spread to other tissues of the body. Treatment is by surgical excision and, if further spread has occurred, treatment will become more intense, complicated and almost always unsuccessful. This is why an early visit to your doctor is strongly advised.

Squamous cell carcinoma (SCC)

SCC has a high rate of cure when treated at an early stage. This type of skin cancer appears as a raised scaly solid nodule and occurs mainly in older people. It grows quickly and can double in size in a few months. Left untreated, it turns into a red ulcerated lump that does not heal. It develops most on areas that have been exposed to the sun, such as the face, neck, back of hands, upper chest or back. SCC is linked to constant exposure to the sun over many years but can also be caused by certain substances used in manufacturing and industry.

Basal cell carcinoma (BCC – rodent ulcer)

This most common cancer is found mainly in people over the age of 60. The most common variety appears as a bump or nodule and is slow growing. It may first appear translucent but if left untreated develops a raised, pearly border. Over a period of time it becomes larger, developing in the centre to an ulcer that does not heal. BCC usually affects the inner corner of the eyes and the area around the nose, and other parts of the skin of the face. Other varieties of BCC present different characteristics and medical advice should always be sought.

Birth marks

Q. *Why do some people get birth marks?*

A. I am not sure why birth marks appear, but they are found on some babies when they are born or they show up in the first few weeks of life. A **congenital naevus** or mole is one type of birthmark that is present at birth. The common type is the **vascular birthmark**, where vessels have gathered closely together just under the surface of the skin. **Macular stains** are another common type of birthmark. These can also be referred to as 'salmon' marks because of their colour. Faint red marks appear anywhere on the body. The eyelids, forehead and the back of the neck are common areas. These stains will often disappear before a child goes to school. However, the ones on the back of the neck last longer. The **strawberry mark** is where the growth is close to the surface of the skin showing a reddish strawberry colour. This will disappear before adult life. **Port wine stains** are lifelong vascular birthmarks that affect a small percentage of children born each year. They are flat, with colours ranging from pink through to dark purple, and are most common on the face, neck, arms and legs. Port wine stains can have complications if they are on the face near the eyelids or forehead. The major disability is the appearance of these stains which can be disfiguring.

Cosmetically

Makeup to cover the stain may help.

Medically

Laser treatment has really shown various degrees of success in removing port wine stains. Seek medical advice if the mark or stain needs to be removed.

Blackheads

Q. *What causes blackheads on the nose and chin?*

A. The nose, chin and forehead are part of the T-zone area where most oil glands are active. Oil (sebum) becomes trapped in the pores of the skin. Oxidation takes place and this causes the oil to turn black. The term for blackheads is 'comedones'. People with oily skins are more prone to have blackheads. The most common place I have found blackheads on older women is between the grooves on each side of the nose and on the tip of the nose.

Q. *What can I do to get rid of blackheads?*

A. First of all, a good diet will help reduce the occurrence of blackheads. Eating the right kinds of food will help reduce oil in the skin, increase good moisture and help the production of new skin cells. Eat plenty of fresh fruit and vegetables and the 'good fats' as in avocados, nuts, olives. Avoid saturated fats and minimize the intake of carbohydrates.

Cosmetically

Develop a daily cleansing routine using cosmetics designed to help remove blackheads. Exfoliate two to three times weekly to help remove any dead skin cells. A green clay mask with lavender oil and infusion once a week will help remove blackheads. Never force the blackheads out of the pore by squeezing either manually or by using an instrument. Squeezing can cause permanent damage to the pores which can lead to scarring, infections, open pores, large spots, pimples and cysts.

Alternatives

These may include herbal remedies, nutrition, aromatherapy and face reflexology.

Broken capillaries

Q. *What causes broken capillaries?*

A. As the skin thins, it becomes more vulnerable to the elements, such as sunshine, and to exposure to central heating, air conditioning, industrial chemicals, harsh weather (extreme cold or heat), neglect in skin protection, or injury. Internal factors which may cause broken capillaries are medication, spicy foods, flushed skin, hormonal changes, stress, hot drinks, alcohol and cigarette smoke. Dilated capillaries on a fine skin texture assume a general vascular appearance, often affecting large areas of the face. The skin responds to any stimulation and permanent dilated vessels are apparent especially on the upper cheeks and nose. The fineness of the skin and its general sensitivity give guidance as to the probability of split capillary formation and limit the range of possible treatments. Spider Naevus (telangiectatic angiomas) are smaller capillaries radiating from a central capillary like the legs of a spider. It is also called a 'broken vein' and may be isolated or in an area of vascular skin such as the cheeks. This problem usually develops in adult life and is commonly found in the face, particularly on the upper cheek and eye areas.

Cosmetically

The use of creams for sensitive skin may be appropriate; stimulation such as exfoliation and excessive massage treatments need to be used with caution, or not at all.

Medically

Laser treatment has been known to be successful in repair work of broken capillaries.

Bruises

Q. *Why do some people bruise more easily than others?*

A. A bruise is caused by a haemorrhage into the tissues from ruptured blood vessels beneath the skin surface, without the skin itself being broken. This is also referred to as a contusion. As the skin thins, and fat tissue loses its resilience and decreases, blood vessels in the skin appear more visible and prominent as they enlarge, becoming vulnerable to any external injury. This is why people after middle years, older people, especially women, bruise easily. Other factors that can cause bruising are blood disorders, blood thinning medications, other medications (internal and topical), injury, intravenous injections and catheters, and heavy external pressure to the skin and muscle tissue. Frail older persons are very prone to bruising, especially in areas of a bony prominence (e.g. the hips, knees, ankles, elbows and cheeks). Bruising can easily occur in medically frail people who are immobile. Crossing of ankles or sliding down in a bed can cause a bruise and, should a skin lesion occur with bruising, it can lead to a bed sore (Decubitus ulcer) if left unattended.

Cosmetically

Do not apply any cosmetic to a bruised area nor any force or pressure.

Medically

For severe bruising, seek medical advice.

Q. *What are cherry angiomas?*

A. These are harmless, small red bumps or spots created by dilated blood vessels. They are common and can be seen on any part of the body. They can appear on the skin from teen years but more commonly from middle age onwards.

Cosmetically

No harm will occur with cosmetic application. Makeup camouflage can be useful for spots on the face.

Medically

These can be removed by cautery or laser treatment.

Pregnancy

Q. *What causes brown marks to appear on the skin during pregnancy?*

A. Hormonal changes brought about by pregnancy are common causes for brown marks. These marks (chloasma) fade after pregnancy. They can also appear on women who are taking the contraceptive pill and in women who are having hormonal treatment during the menopause. Chloasma is a benign skin condition that has a dark brown appearance and is often found on the face and other parts of the body that are exposed to the sun.

Cosmetically

Use a sunscreen and moisture cream with an SPF 30 and take protection from the sun.

Medically

Any topical medications to be used during pregnancy should be discussed with a health care practitioner before use.

Alternatives

Reflexology, face reflexology, aromatherapy, herbal remedies, flower remedies.

During pregnancy, it is wise to seek medical advice before using alternative therapies.

Cold sores

Q. *Why are some people more prone to cold sores than others?*

A. A cold sore is due to a virus (herpes simplex). The virus lies dormant in cells and can be triggered by cold (hence the name). Strong sunlight, too much stress, being run down, are other factors that trigger cold sores. Many people develop a natural immunity to the virus and never suffer from a cold sore, while in others, cold sores occur frequently, especially in winter. The infection is easily spread to another person by sharing products such as lipsticks, lip pencils, by drinking from another person's cup or water bottle and by body contact, especially if the infection is at its most active stage when the sores are filled with fluid.

Cosmetically

Do not apply any cosmetic product over a cold sore unless it has some medicinal properties that are suited to calm inflamed lesions. Do not go for any beauty facial treatment while the cold sore is inflamed.

Medically

Topical creams purchased from a pharmacist may help to treat cold sores and inflammation.

Alternatives

Herbal remedies, aromatherapy and nutritious diet may be of benefit.

Whiteheads

Q. *What are whiteheads and what causes them to appear?*

A. Whiteheads (milia) can appear singularly or in clusters on any part of the body but more on the face, arms and back. Whiteheads are more inclined to accumulate in clusters on people with oily skins. They occur when the dead skin cells accumulate with other material inside the follicles and block the pores. The trapped material can remain inside a follicle for a long time or it can disperse leaving no blemishes or scars, providing that the white-heads have not been squeezed.

Cosmetically

Small recently-formed whiteheads can be removed with the help of a qualified beauty therapist.

Medically

The hard large lumps that have been on the skin for a long time are best treated either through laser treatment or by a medical practitioner such as a dermatologist.

Pimples

Q. *Why do pimples occur if you do not have acne or oily skin?*

A. A tender red lump (papule or blind pimple) forms on the surface of the skin. As it gets larger, the follicle ruptures and spills its infectious contents of dead skin cells into the surrounding skin. White blood cells enter the area to attack this material, forming pus, and a pimple (pustule) results. A cyst forms when the inflam-mation spreads deep within the skin. Possible causes may be the use of contaminated products, poor hygiene procedures, friction on the skin by wearing clothes too tight, a bacterial infection, or a hormonal imbalance.

Cosmetically

Use an antibacterial cream to help combat the spread of pustules. Facials with a beauty therapist will benefit troublesome skin.

Medically

For severe cases, seek medical advice.

Alternatives

These may include nutrition, herbal remedies, face reflexology and massage.

Warts

Q. *Is it true that if you put milk thistle on a wart it will disappear?*

A. Over the years I have heard a few myths about how to get rid of warts. I have heard of milk thistle, though have never tried it. A wart will disappear over a period of time and this can take a lot of patience. Warts are contagious (but harmless) skin growths that can appear on any part of the body, mostly affecting the hands, face and feet. There are various types of warts and they affect only the epidermis. They spread through direct contact from one part of the body to another. A wart is due to a virus that invades the skin cells, causing them to multiply quickly, leading to a dry lump on the surface.

Medically

Warts can be removed by a medical practitioner using cryo-surgery or electrocautery, which burns away the skin.

Q. *What are these small wart-like tags on the neck?*

A. These are called skin tags (fibroepithelial polyps). They look like little tags attached to the skin (hence the name skin tags). Skin tags are small, brown to a light brown or flesh colour, and mainly grow on the neck, under the arms, in the groin and on eyelids. They affect middle-aged to older persons and are very common.

The cause is unknown, but they are often found in overweight people, especially women.

Q. *These rough sores on the face won't heal. What are they?*

A. The scaly patches are known as Actinic keratosis. These rough red scaly patches appear like warts and occur mainly on the face, neck, hands or forearms as a result of constant exposure to the sun in early life. They are more common in older persons who have been exposed to the sun. The sores form a crust; the crust falls off and then re-forms. They do not heal normally. If left untreated, they may have the potential to become cancerous. A cutaneous horn which produces a hard yellowish, dry, scaly horny nodule may develop in actinic keratosis. These horny lesions are unsightly and can become a nuisance. Older people are often affected with a cutaneous horn which I have seen grow from the side of the face (near the temples) and sides and backs of the hand.

Cosmetically

Cosmetic use is acceptable though you should use creams and cleansers lightly. When applying, be careful not to pull off sores and cause bleeding.

Medically

Some medical practitioners may suggest to use keratolytic agents urea or salicylic creams and to keep them well moisturized and protect from the sun. They can be removed if necessary.

Psoriasis

Q. *What causes psoriasis?*

A. There is no known cause for psoriasis, however there are a number of precipitating factors which are associated with the disorder, such as trauma to the epidermis and dermis, infection, drugs, sunlight, stress. Psoriasis is a chronic non-infectious inflammatory skin disorder which appears as red to silvery scaly plaques, involving the elbows, knees, scalp, hair margin or sacrum. It occurs as a result of an imbalance in the turnover of skin cells where growth is much faster than for normal skin. Other forms of psoriasis that show up on the skin include drop-like lesions that appear on the back and limbs and are referred to as 'Guttae'. Psoriasis that affects the axillae and sub-mammary areas is known as flexural psoriasis. Palmoplantar pustulosis is a localized variant of psoriasis that occurs on the sole of the foot and palms of the hands. The most severe form of psoriasis which can be life-threatening is Generalized pustular psoriasis. It is an acute form that can be very painful. Sore-like lesions occur with yellowish pustules that develop on very red skin.

Cosmetically

For mild cases of psoriasis, some moisture creams such as sorbolene or night creams may be suitable. Light cleansing and a gentle facial massage may be of benefit for some people.

Medically

This disorder is treated with medicated topical creams. Severe psoriasis is treated under the supervision of a medical person as the individual may require oral medications as well as medicated topical creams.

Alternatives

Essential oils (jojoba, avocado, carrot, calendula, almond) may help soothe irritated skin in mild psoriasis. For mild cases, massage, reflexology, Bowen massage, face reflexology and flower remedies may also be of benefit.

Varicose veins

Q. *What causes varicose veins to appear?*

A. Varicose veins show as enlarged leg veins that appear blue, streaky and patchy with a network of smaller veins. Some have a nodule appearance like hard raised lumps on the legs. The veins become twisted or swollen when blood, returning to the heart against gravity, flows back down the veins because the valves in the veins are faulty or absent. The cause of varicose veins is a genetic lack of one-way valves in the veins of the lower limbs. Pregnancy and professions where people spend a lot of time standing, coupled with the genetic background, give rise to this condition.

Varicose ulcers occur as late development of varicose veins and are found more commonly in the middle aged and onwards. This condition is due to skin breakdown following blood flow stasis or stagnation. Early symptoms are redness and itchiness followed by skin breakdown and ulcer formation.

Medically

Topical medicated creams are available from your local pharmacist. Surgery may be an option for some individuals who have a severe form of varicose veins. Regular exercise of a non-jarring type is beneficial. Keep the legs elevated when at rest. Surgical stockings should also be worn.

Alternatives

For varicose veins, soak the legs in a herbal bath to help soothe tired aching legs. Place a muslin bag filled with 3 tbs of chamomile flowers and 3 tbs of calendula flowers, over the hot water while running the bath. Exercise regularly to help improve circulation. Rest legs while raising them up on a cushion or similar. A good healthy diet and exercise are important to help combat sluggish circulation.

White patches

Q. *What causes white patches on the skin?*

A. This is a loss of pigmentation where the pigment-producing cells have been damaged. This disorder is called 'vitiligo'. The colour in the skin ranges from either white or pink resembling spots, patches or marks. The exact cause of vitiligo is unknown but it is thought to be genetic and can run in families. Other causes may be chemical, injury, illness, hormonal disorder, burns and stress. There is no cure for this condition.

Cosmetically
Camouflage makeup can help to disguise the patches.

Medically
Treatment is difficult, but some medications may stop the patches from spreading in early stages. Keep out of sunlight, as this can make the condition worse.

Useful websites

The websites listed below are current at the time of my research on 30 June 2008 before publication.

Nevus Outreach Inc. (2007) Melanocytic Naevi
www.nevus.org

National Psoriasis Foundation (2008) Psoriasis
www.psoriasis.org

The Cancer Council Victoria (June 2008) Skin Cancer
www.sunsmart.com.au

American Academy of Dermatology (2008) Skin Disorders
www.aad.org

Medline Plus (June 2008) Skin Ageing
www.nlm.nih.gov/medlineplus/skinaging.html

Glossary

Actinic
Produced by chemically active rays beyond the violet end of the light spectrum.

Allergen
A substance such as foods, plants, industrial chemicals capable of inducing an allergy or hypersensitivity.

Angioma
Benign tumour, made up of blood or lymph vessels.

Antibody
A blood protein produced in response to and then counteracting antigens.

Antigen
Foreign substance (toxin) which causes the body to produce antibodies.

Axillae
Under the arms.

Benign
Not malignant. Favourable for recovery.

Blemishes
Combination of skin marks, spots, disorders that appear on, or show through, the skin.

Capillaries
Small blood vessels branching from and connecting arterioles to venules.

Catheter
A tubular flexible instrument passed through, body channels for withdrawal of fluids, or introduction of fluids into a body cavity.

Cautery
The application of a caustic agent, a hot instrument, an electric current, or another agent to destroy tissue.

Comedone
Blackhead.

Congenital
Present at and existing from the time of birth.

Contusion
Injury to tissues without breakage of the skin such as a bruise.

Cutaneous

Relating to the skin, and to the cuticles.

Dander

Small scales (or skin flakes) from the hair of animals and feathers of birds. May be the cause of allergy in sensitive persons.

Decubitus ulcer

Bed sore or pressure sore.

Dermatologist

A medical person who specializes in treating skin diseases and disorders.

Diagnose

To identify symptoms, disease, or an illness.

Distension

Swelling by pressure from within.

Electrocautery

Cauterization of tissue by means of an electrode that consists of metal such as a wire held in a holder, and heated by either direct or alternating currents.

Face reflexology

A complementary therapy that aids in the body's healing by gentle stimulation of the reflexes on the face. Helps to tone the muscles, improve circulation, relieve stress, improve sinus problems, relieve headache pain, aid in digestion and expel impurities from the skin.

Facial

A beauty treatment that involves the face, neck, and sometimes the décolletage, arms and shoulders. Techniques include the cleansing of the skin, exfoliation, face massage, face mask and skin analysis.

Flower remedies

Plants are floated in pure water in the sunlight, energizing the water with their molecular imprint. This has led to the development of incorporating many flowers including those from, for example, the tea-tree bush. These remedies have properties for the relief of ailments and the treatment of emotions which can trigger physical conditions.

Intravenous   Administration of fluids via a vein.

Irritant   An agent that causes irritation.

Laser   A device that generates an intense beam of coherent light, or other electromagnetic radiation, in one direction (light amplification by stimulated emission of radiation) used as a tool in surgery, in diagnosis and in physiological studies.

Lesion   A wound or injury creating a pathological change in the tissue.

Macula   A small spot perceptibly different in colour from the surrounding tissue.

Mammary   Relating to the breast.

Massage   A therapeutic body therapy that incorporates skilled touch and stroke techniques to help promote efficiency in the body's systems, in turn enhancing the functioning of the entire person.

Medically frail   An ill person dependent on full care for their medical and physical welfare.

Menopause   Permanent cessation of the menses. Termination of the menstrual period or 'change of life'. A phase in life in which a woman passes from the reproductive to the non-reproductive phase.

Moles   Small permanent dark raised spots that appear on the skin.

Necrolysis   Separation or exfoliation of necrotic tissue.

Nevus (nevi)   Benign localized overgrowth of melanin forming cells arising in the skin early in life.

Nodule   A small solid mass of tissue in the form of a swelling, knot or protuberance.

Oedema   An accumulation of excessive amount of watery fluid in cells, tissues or serous cavities.

Oestrogen   Female sex hormone developing and maintaining female characteristics of the body.

Palmoplantar warts   These are epidermal tumours that appear on the palm of the hand or sole of the foot and are caused by a virus.

Polyps   Overgrowth of normal tissue. A growth protruding from a mucous membrane. Polyps may be attached to a thin stalk such as skin tags. These are known as pedunculated polyps. Broad flat polyps are known as sessile polyps.

Reflexology   A powerful therapy that has the ability to work the circulatory systems and helps stimulate the body's own healing power to maintain health and well-being. It involves the stimulation of pressure points on the feet, hands or face that correspond to the glands and organs of the body.

Rhinophyma   A severe form of rosacea involving the lower half of the nose and sometimes spreading to adjacent cheek areas. Usually seen in adult males. Characterized by a thickened, lobulated overgrowth of sebaceous glands and epithelial connective tissue.

Sacrum	Triangular bone of the spine between the two hips.
Sebaceous	Relating to sebum.
Sebum	Oily, fatty secretions of the sebaceous glands.
Serous	Watery substance of a gland or membrane like serum.
Serum	Liquid that separates from a clot when blood coagulates. Watery fluid in animal bodies.
Skin analysis	Diagnosis of the condition of the skin, its texture, colour, type, skin blemishes, disorders, either cosmetically or medically.
Synthesis	Combination of elements into a whole. Artificial production of compounds from their constituents as distinct from extraction from plants.
Telangiectasis	Vascular lesion formed by dilation. A group of small blood vessels.
Ulcer	Open sore on or in the body, often forming pus. Produced by sloughing of necrotic inflammatory tissue.
Vascular	A system of vessels that circulate the blood.
Vessel	Hollow receptacle.

CHAPTER 7

Skin Care and Makeup

Skin cleansing
Facial care for frail older people
Makeup application
The correct colour code
Colour coding for older women
Cosmetic accessories and colour cosmetics
Makeup application tips for older women
Conclusion
Useful websites
Glossary

Skin cleansing

The most important part of skin care is cleansing, especially the face and neck areas, as these are most exposed to the elements and pollution. Through the day, the skin picks up a huge amount of dirt and grime especially in the city. It is important never to leave any makeup on the face while sleeping, as this only adds to pores becoming more clogged by house dust particles settling on the skin along with the stale makeup. Cleansing of the face and neck area should be carried out at least twice daily. The morning's cleanse helps to eliminate any house dust particles and will rejuvenate the skin. The evening's cleanse takes care of daily pollution and stale makeup, refreshing the skin. The skin may need to be cleansed again before an evening social outing. All makeup should be removed and reapplied, if appropriate, after cleansing. The evening cleanse should be carried out at the end of the day before going to bed.

Basic steps to cleanse the skin

1   Use either a clean soft towel, sponge, or disposable cotton pads.

2   Gently wet the face.

3   Apply the cleanser to the palm of your hand or take from a spatula, gently working the cleanser to a light lather over the face.

4   Begin at the neck, chin, and work up over the cheeks to the forehead with circular movements of the hands.

5   Next, work down the nose and into the sides of the nostrils. Move along the top lip line, over the lips (keeping mouth closed) then down to the neck again.

6   Repeat the sequence two to three times but there is no need to add extra cleanser.

7   Rinse off the cleanser either by washing water over the face (this can be done in a shower), by sprinkling water over the face standing at the sink, or use a face cloth, sponge or disposable cotton pads.

8   Pat dry the face and neck using a soft towel.

For foam cleansers, pour a small portion into the palm of your hand and lather before applying to the face. For tube cleansers, place a small drop onto a spatula and place a small dot on each cheek, the forehead, chin, tip of nose and the neck. Work over the face using circular movements. For cream cleansers, use same circular movements. Never use your fingers to remove cream from a jar (see Cosmetic hygiene care, in Chapter 1). Soap cleansers can be used in the same way as foam cleansers.

Toning (Skin freshener)

1   Use a skin freshener to take away any residue left on the skin.

2   Place the freshener onto a light damp cotton wool ball.

3   Pat the skin all over with the cotton wool ball, then gently wipe the areas that hold extra residue from the cleansing.

4   Repeat the use of the skin freshener with a clean cotton ball once more.

5   The face should feel refreshed, cleansed and smooth.

Moisturizing

1   Place the moisture cream, liquid or gel onto a spatula.

2   Dot the moisture cream over the face and neck.

3   Use circular movements to absorb the moisture cream into the skin.

4   A tinted moisture cream with an SPF may be added for day wear.

Facial exfoliation

Exfoliant creams or liquids are cosmetics that contain abrasive material to help remove dead skin cells from the surface of the skin and prevent the pores from becoming blocked. Soft abrasive sponges or brushes are suitable for use when exfoliating the skin. If the skin is too sensitive to apply a brush or an abrasive sponge, gently massage the cream over the skin in a circular motion using your fingers and hands. Do not work too long in one area as this can cause the skin to redden, especially if it is sensitive. Wash the cream or liquid off and pat dry. Once or twice weekly is enough for a facial exfoliation for most skin types but people with very oily skin may need to exfoliate more often.

Face mask

For most skin types, a weekly facial mask is probably sufficient. The function of a mask is to cleanse the skin deep down into the pores, ridding it of grime, blackheads and dead skin cells, leaving it feeling refreshed, smooth and clean. Before applying a mask, make sure the face has been cleansed. Follow instructions from the leaflet with your mask product and apply as directed. Most masks for the home user are easy to apply. A clay mask, for instance, can be mixed with water or a herbal infusion, with a drop of essential oil (see Herbal Remedies and Essential Oils, Chapter 3). Using a soft brush, apply the mask, starting at the forehead with upward strokes from the brow line to the hair line along the forehead finishing at the end of the brow line to centre of outer eye (do not go too close to the eyes). Next, cover the cheek area moving towards the jaw line, meeting up around the eye area to the end of the line where you finished off at the forehead. This makes a complete circle around the eye area. Brush down the nose from the centre of the brows then extend over the nostril folds. Brush down and out along the top lip line but do not cover lips, and extend towards the outer curve of the lips. From the bottom lip line, brush down over the chin. Brush in a circular movement across the neck, following the grooves and creases. Make sure you leave the eye area, nostrils and mouth free from mask application. Leave the mask to dry for about 15–20 minutes, rinse off the mask and then moisturize the face and neck. Some masks may need to stay on longer. While the mask is setting on the face and neck, adding herbally infused eye pads to the eyes will have a soothing effect. (See Formula for clay mask, Chapter 3).

Facial care for frail older people

Frail older persons will be able to cope with a cleansing routine but it would be best not to use a face cloth if the skin is very sensitive. A sponge or disposable cotton pad would be suitable. It is also best not to overstimulate the skin and circulation, therefore possibly one cleansing sequence would be enough. For the carer giving the facial it would be easier to stand behind the person receiving the treatment and work over the face starting from the neck upwards. This can be done if the person is sitting in a chair or (better for the carer) if the person is lying on the bed and the bed end can extend or be taken out, creating more room. Be careful when washing around the eyes and over the mouth. It would be best to wash these areas first before the full cleansing treatment commences. If the frail person has body fluids leaking from the eyes, nose, mouth or ears, use disposable gloves for protection.

Makeup application

The disadvantages of wearing makeup

Makeup application is a personal choice; it is not necessary to apply any colour cosmetic to the face if the person is happy to be free from any form of coloured makeup. People with a sensitive skin and those with multiple skin conditions may find colour makeup uncomfortable to wear. Colour makeup should only be worn for short periods of time. Makeup worn for long periods of time, especially if the skin has not been cleansed in between makeup applications, will end up seeping into and clogging the pores of the skin. This will suffocate the skin's natural moisturizing agent, allowing the excreting oil and sweat to lie beneath the makeup, creating more skin problems. Many minor skin blemishes such as papules, pimples and cysts are caused through neglect, by removing makeup incorrectly and by 'poor' skin cleansing.

The benefits of wearing makeup

For those who like to wear colour makeup, there are some benefits. Makeup has the ability to camouflage unsightly spots, marks, scars and other skin imperfections. It can accentuate the best features, add tone and colour to the complexion and restore confidence by helping a person to feel and look good.

Common makeup mistakes

The most common mistakes to avoid in makeup application are as follows:

Foundation

The most frequent mistake is to use the wrong tone, which does not match the natural skin colour. The foundation can be applied too heavily and unevenly. Sometimes it can look like a mask. Foundation can also look blotchy.

Blushers or rouge

The main error here is wearing the wrong colour. The blusher looks too heavy and makes the face look flushed with pink tones or a dark dirty colour with heavy yellow undertones. Blusher is either applied in a thin line over the cheek bone or in a round blob on the cheeks with too much in one area.

Powder

This can also be applied too heavily and unevenly causing caking of the makeup. It may also be the wrong colour.

Eye shadow

The colours can be too heavy and, if applied wrongly over the eyelids and around the eyes, can give an appearance of receding eyes, or 'panda eyes'. If too many pink tones are applied this can give an appearance of a 'bruised' look.

Eye liners and eye pencils

Eye liners can be applied too heavily making the eyes look very small. Liquid eye liners will smudge if incorrectly applied. Eye pencils are used for eye liners and eyebrows. Some women who have little eyebrow hair will often draw a thick pencil line across the brows which will give a 'clown' look or a look of surprise. Often the colour of the pencilled brows will not match the hair colour, which draws attention to the lines.

Mascara

This can be applied too thickly, making the eyes look heavy and causing the mascara to clog. The eyelashes may stick together, giving an uneven appearance.

Lipstick

The most common problem is 'bleeding lipstick' and older women are prone to this problem. This happens when the lips have decreased in size and the skin around the lips has many folds which become little grooves for the lipstick to seep into. Other problems are choosing the wrong coloured lipstick and applying the lipstick too thickly and unevenly along the lip line. Lipstick that rubs onto the teeth is also a problem as is lipstick applied in the middle of lips, not covering the full lip line, and showing a 'cupid' or 'heart shape' look.

Stuck in the 'era' of yesterday

Some middle-aged and older women are comfortable wearing makeup the way they have worn it since their youth. They will continue to use the same colours, the same techniques of makeup application and the same colour foundation, as this makes them feel and look good. New trends and the introduction of new colours and makeup techniques are often difficult for some of these women to embrace.

In my experience I have found that some women, even though they liked the 'new' look of being fashionable, found it difficult to change. They said they were much happier with what they were used to, even though they knew that some of the new colours or techniques suited them best. The important issue here is never to try to change a person when they are not ready. As a carer, your aim would be to apply makeup on the person in care, in the way they prefer.

The correct colour code

Q. *How do you know what makeup suits a particular skin tone and hair colour?*

A. This can be a problem for many women. Knowing what colour best suits them is difficult for those who are not familiar with makeup techniques. I have set out below a basic formula for most skin types and tones, as a guide that may help the home user. However, an individual may need to experiment with certain colours before they feel comfortable.

For people of Caucasian origin

Cool tone look

Hair colour may range from blonde to dark blonde, dark hair or red hair. Complexion (skin tone) may look pale to pink, ivory 'English rose' complexion, or 'China doll'. This skin type will burn easily in the sun so would probably need a protection of SPF 30 or 30+. Eye shadow colours that would suit this colouring are usually pale pastel colours. Younger people can wear shimmery and liquid colours. People from middle years onwards would benefit from using matt colours. Grey-blue, to silver, lilac would suit some older women. Foundations should have pink or ivory undertones. Blushers or rouge may be in soft pinks. Red-haired people can wear soft peachy pinks, or if the skin is very pale it may not be necessary to apply any blusher or rouge.

Older women may find it best to use powdered blushers because of their matt texture and natural look. Rouge or cream-based blushers can emphasize creases and folds on the face of a mature skin.

Warm tone look

Hair may be golden warm blonde, dark blonde, mid to dark brown, or orange-red to a warm red hue. The complexion may look warm to a light tan hue, with yellow undertones, and the skin type may tan lightly. You would possibly need an SPF 25+. The tint of eye shadow that may suit this colouring would be peach, soft browns or red-browns. Red-haired people can wear lilacs, pale mauves or wine-toned hues. Foundations with yellow undertones would probably suit this skin type. Blushers in peach, tawny peach, or rosy browns would be suitable. Red-haired people may find peach to light browns best for their skin tone.

People of Mediterranean or Eastern Indian origin

Women with a darker complexion may find light application of colour makeup is sufficient to enhance their skin and features. Most are fortunate to inherit beautiful dark features in their eyelashes and brows along with larger eyes and fuller lips.

Dark hair and olive skin

This skin type does not burn easily and an SPF 15+ would possibly be suitable. The skin can become sensitive to the sun's rays, so sun protection is necessary. Eye shadow colours that may enhance the eyes are in gold, bronze, browns, plums and taupe. Foundations vary in yellow undertones, copper, tan to dark tones. Blushers may be with peach or taupe tones. Lipstick colours that may be suitable are the berries, plums and almonds.

People of Asian origin

Dark brown to blue black hair

Skin tone ranges from an olive complexion with light to dark yellow undertones. Foundations more suitable are the yellow to yellow-tan undertones. Avoid pale pink to orange undertones as they can look ashy and show more like a mask. Some Asian skin types can easily burn in the sun while other types don't. However, Asian skin has a tendency to suffer with sensitivity therefore a daily sunscreen application would be advisable. Use an SPF 15 to 30+. Eye shadow colours that may be suitable are the lilacs, sky blue, pale greens, browns and ivories. Eyeliners in blue-black tones or deep brown (liquid is probably best).* Blushers are best suited in tones of warm pinks or peach.

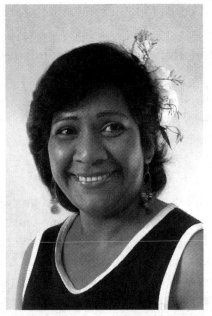

Plate 7.1 The model is wearing a water-based foundation suited for her oily skin. She has been made up for her wedding day and is wearing matt eye shadow colours in lilac, grape and deep pink hues to complement her skin texture and overall look.

---

*   Some Asian women would look best without eyeliner and possibly the eyes would look best with any of the aforementioned eye shadows.

People with dark skin

Black hair with reddish or golden highlights

Skin tone is either pale black or dark black. This type of skin tans easily with very little sun burning.* Eye shadow colours which can enhance the eyes are ivory, brown, lilacs, musky pinks for lighter skin tone. Foundations best suited may be in peach to tan. Blushers could be in a neutral to peach tones. Neutral colours, grape hues and earth tone colours may complement darker skins.

Older women may not need to use blushers or foundations; a tinted moisture cream with powder or a mineral powder would probably be sufficient for a complete coverage.

Colour coding for older women

As a person ages, the colour of their skin tone may change to a lighter or a darker hue and the colour of the hair also changes. Application of makeup needs to be of lighter shades than their skin tone and complemented with a matt finish. Soft pastel colours are more suitable as any dark colours will only add or accentuate creases and furrows. Cream-based cosmetics will only highlight wrinkles and creases, so they are best avoided. A matt finish makeover is a better option as it gives a soft flattering look. The hair of Caucasian women shows either a light brown, to a grey or white colour. If the skin tone is cool, eye shadow colours best suited may be a cocoa brown or grey, silver, pale pink or a champagne highlighter. Blushers of a soft plum or dusty rose will look best for women with a warm skin tone where the hair shows an ash brown, grey or white, and eye shadows that complement are the neutrals, pink-browns, greys, plums, and peachy pinks. Blushers are either natural or neutral colours.

***

* Wearing sunscreen can help to diminish hyperpigmentation and scarring when acne or a rash fades.

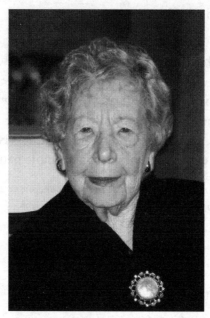

Plate 7.2 The model is wearing a light makeup application.

Darker-skinned people of other origins may be able to continue using the same colours as before, except for the use of lighter shades of eye shadows. Eye shadow powder instead of eye liners and a softer coloured lipstick would be more suitable. A blusher may not be necessary for makeup application, depending on the skin condition.

Older people would probably need a higher SPF due to drying and thinning of the skin, coupled with sensitivity. Tinted moisturizers for day wear are a better alternative than the use of a foundation for frail women of all origins. Some concealers may help to disguise minor blemishes.

Q. *Does eye colour have anything to do with choosing the correct colour code?*

A. Yes, it does help. You do not have to keep to one or two colours because of eye colour. There are many different coloured palettes of eye shadow on the market today. You can explore and practise to find what suits a person best, following the basic guidelines of skin type and hair colour. An easier option would be to consult a beauty therapist or makeup artist. This is money well spent. A client would be shown what colours best suit her, where to accentuate her best features, how to apply sensible and easy techniques for makeup application. The therapist will also be able to advise on 'classic' and 'signature' colours.

Q. *What is the correct way of applying foundation?*

A. Firstly, make sure that the skin is moist. Use a damp sponge wedge from which all excess water has been squeezed out. When taking the foundation from a tube or jar, use a spatula and place enough liquid or cream to cover the face. (A dot the size of your thumb nail would probably be enough.) Apply sparingly at first, and then add more if necessary. You can either apply the foundation in dots over the face and then blend it in with the sponge wedge or directly place the foundation from a spatula onto the sponge. Start to apply from the centre of the face (the T-zone area) and extend outwards over the cheeks, and chin and down towards the neck, making sure the foundation blends in well, leaving no streaky marks. If the hair is worn up away from the ears, it helps to apply a little foundation over the bottom ear lobes: this gives a natural look to the whole face. Foundation should blend well with the skin tone. If it is too light, or too dark, then it is not the correct colour. Foundation should also complement the client's skin tone and give the appearance that it is the natural skin tone colour. If the foundation is applied too heavily, it will look as if the person is wearing a mask. I find that using the sponge wedge is the easiest way to apply foundation.

Q. *What are the benefits of wearing face powder and what is the correct way of applying it?*

A. The benefit of wearing face powder is that it gives a good coverage over the face and neck by setting the foundation and colour makeup and keeping it in place a lot longer. Powder also gives a super-smooth sheen to the skin with or without the foundation. Powder absorbs oil from the skin, and helps prevent shiny patches. Loose powders are best for setting makeup. Once the foundation is applied, dip a powder puff or cotton pad into the powder and blot the powder over the face, especially the eye and lip areas. This will set the eye shadow and lipstick, helping it last longer. The face may look a bit blotchy. Using a large powder brush, brush downward strokes all over the face and neck, making sure you blend the powder evenly over the skin, eyes and lips. The face should look natural with no blotches or streaks, and is now ready for the coloured makeup.

Q. *Should concealers be applied before or after foundation?*

A. Concealers are used to conceal blemishes, shadows, scars, red veins and spots. When choosing a concealer, look for a colour nearest to that of the client's skin. There has always been a bit of controversy as to whether a concealer should be used before or after foundation. Basically this depends on the type of concealer to be used. Coloured cream concealers such as green, mauve and yellow have been used in the past to camouflage blemishes before applying foundation. Over the years, I have found these cream colours to be useless as they will often show through the foundation and provide very little benefit. Recently I have found liquid concealer to be more beneficial when used after the application of foundation and before powder. The thicker cream-based concealers are best used before application of a foundation. Use a small brush to apply a liquid concealer over the blemished area and blend with the foundation. Sponge applicators are most suitable for cream-based concealers. Add powder after the concealer and foundation, as the powder will help to set them both.

Older women may require a lighter concealer, as sometimes ageing skin grooves are too dark, especially around the eyes and lip area. Adding dark concealer will only give the appearance of deeper furrows and accentuate these areas.

Q. *How should a blusher be applied?*

A. Powder blushers are applied over foundation and powder. Cream-based blushers and rouge are applied before powder application. A blusher can be applied either before eye shadow or at the end of the makeup application. (I find it easier to apply powdered blusher at the end of eye shadow application. This makes it easier to judge how much depth of colour is needed, taking into consideration the colour hues used over the eye areas.) You should dust over powder blusher compact with a large soft brush and tap the handle to get rid of excess blusher. Begin the colour on the fullest part of the cheeks directly below the centre of the eyes, in line with the iris. Ask the person to smile, as this helps to make the cheek bones stand out and it is easier to see where the blusher should be. Blush over the cheekbones up towards the temples, but not as far as the temples or as far down as the jaw line. Blend well and don't leave a definite line. If you have applied too much blusher, add powder over the top until you get the colour texture you want. The idea of using a blusher is to put colour back into the cheeks where natural blushing should occur. Cream blushers can be applied with fingers or a foundation wedge sponge, blending well before the application of powder. (I prefer to use the wedged sponge, as it makes application easier.)

Powdered blushers are best for older women. Cream colour cosmetics will only accentuate lines and furrows. Women with a flushed complexion or women with a pinkish skin tone may not need to use any form of blusher.

Q. *How do you stop mascara from smudging the skin?*

A. First of all, make sure the eye area and eyelashes are powdered and blended. Your mascara wand should be clean and moist, and hold enough mascara for application to each set of lashes. Place a small folded piece of tissue under the eye, apply mascara to lower bottom lashes first, then blink a few times. This will get rid of the excess mascara which will fall onto the tissue. Next apply mascara to the top lashes by brushing downwards first, then underneath the lashes and upwards. Repeat blinking as before. Allow lashes to dry then apply another coat if necessary. (Some people will often place mascara on the top lashes before the bottom lashes. It really is a matter of choice.) Clean your mascara wand before placing it back in the container. Another option is to use disposable mascara wands. This will save the main mascara wand from becoming clogged and protect the mascara from drying out when it is exposed to air. Once the mascara has become dried, throw it away and purchase a new mascara case and wand.

Q. *How much eye shadow should be used at one time?*

A. This is optional. If a person is dressing up for a special occasion or having a photographic portrait taken, they may need a few extra colours to blend in with their overall look. However, for an everyday look, they may need only one to two shadows with perhaps a touch of coloured highlighting or shading hue. If you are not going to use a foundation, it is still a good idea to powder the eyelid as a base to hold the colour.

Using an eye sponge applicator, sweep a neutral eye colour over the eyelids. Work up to the eyebrow line to give a balanced overall look. Using a fresh eye applicator, apply a darker shade of colour along the socket line of the eyes. Use another brush over the top of the dark colour to blend and remove any harsh edges. You may like to leave this as it is, or add more of the light colour to the eyelid. You can, if desired, add another colour to blend with the previous two colours. Mascara can be applied if the client does not want to wear eye liner. Eye liner should be applied before mascara.

Older women would possibly need only two light shades of shadow. Wearing mascara could be difficult for some, having very few eyelashes, eye blemishes, eye disorders or poor eye movement control. Eye shadow can compensate as an eye liner and eyebrow shade, where pencils and eye liners are contraindicated.

Q. *What is the best method for putting a pencil line across the brow?*

A. First follow the natural eyebrow line (see Steps to shaping the eyebrows, in Chapter 4). The eyebrow hairs are generally made up of more than one colour, therefore it is best to work with two coloured pencils which blend well with the client's natural hair colour. For example, if the eyebrows are brown with a touch of grey, then use both brown and grey pencils. Use the brown pencil first as this is the main colour of the brows, and then blend the grey pencil colour next. Draw across the brow line in a feather fashion, following the brow hair line. Do not make a straight line as this will only look artificial. Once the line has been drawn, use a soft sponge pencil or cotton bud to blend the colours, giving a natural look to the brows.

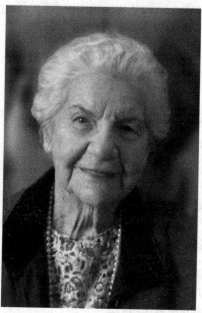

Plate 7.3 The model is wearing day makeup after having her eyebrows shaped and coloured.

Q. *How do I stop lipstick from bleeding into lip lines and getting onto teeth?*

A. Blot the lips with foundation and powder. Using a lip liner (pencils are best) draw along the lip lines of the bottom and top lips. If the lips are too full, bring the line in towards the centre of the lips just a little above the lip line. If the lips are too thin, then extend out a little towards the chin just a little over the bottom lip line. Do the same, extending over the lip line towards the nose, for the top lip. Once the lines have been marked out, you may like to fill in the lips with the pencil liner, or leave the lip lines as they are. Filling in the lips with lip liner will help the lipstick to stay on longer and give another tone of colour. With a lip brush, paint the lips with the lip colour. Blot lips with a tissue to remove excess lipstick. Powder lips and then remove any excess powder. Repeat this sequence two to three times as this will keep the lipstick on the lips for a longer period. When the last application of lipstick is applied, the client should put their index finger in their mouth and place their lips around their finger and press lips down on it. A lipstick circle will show around the finger. This method prevents the lipstick from sticking to the teeth.

Cosmetic accessories and colour cosmetics

Cosmetic accessories

When applying makeup, it is best to have the right tools for the right application. Makeup kits that contain all accessories are easily purchased in department stores and supermarkets at reasonable prices. To understand what tools are used for which cosmetic, the list is as follows:

Makeup sponges Wedged or round shapes for applying foundation. Other shaped sponges are used to apply cream-based cosmetics or as blending accessories.

Powder brush This should be large and soft.

Blusher brush A medium soft brush. Some blusher palettes come with a small blusher brush. These are not as good as the larger soft brushes which give a smooth 'overall' blended look.

Eye shadow brushes These are brushes with a round sponge at the end of the applicator and are used especially for applying shadow. At the other end of the applicator is a brush end that is used for blending. These applicators can be sold singly without the brush at the end.

Powder puff This comes with compact powder. It is used to blot powder over the face but is not as good as the large blusher brushes for smooth blending. Cotton wool pads are a good alternative for a powder puff. Powder puffs are best used for day wear when makeup needs a slight touch-up, and to stop skin-shine caused by the natural oils in the skin.

Eyelash comb and brush One end of the applicator has the brush, the other end a comb, used to comb eyebrows into shape. The eyebrow comb can also be used to comb up eyelashes. The brush can be used to blend pencil or eye shadow colour onto the brows.

Lip brush Used for the application of lipstick.

Disposables These are used for makeup application and hair removal and may be cotton pads, cotton buds, cotton balls, tissues, nail files, cuticle sticks, cotton makeup pads, wax strips, sponges, lip brushes, mascara wands and spatulas.

Colour cosmetics

Concealers Concealers come in liquids, creams, lipstick tubes and stick concealers. Stick concealers are easy to apply. Simply stroke them on to the blemished area and blend with your fingers. Wipe the tube with a tissue when finished. Cream concealers come in either a tube or a palette container with a sponge. Some of these concealers are thicker than others and are good for camouflaging blemishes. Cream concealers are best for application before using powder. Liquid concealers come in a tube and are easy to apply. Just put a small dot of concealer onto a spatula and use a fine brush to dot the concealer over the blemished area, and then blend into the foundation.

Foundation This is used as a base for makeup application. A tinted moisturizer is a form of foundation containing a mixture of moisture cream and a touch of foundation with an SPF. Tinted moisturizers are ideal to wear as a protection for the face and as a substitute for heavier foundations. Liquid foundations come in tubes or bottles and they suit most skin types. Those that are water-based are more suitable for oily skins. They can also be used for other skin types but not for very dry skins. Cream foundations come in palettes or small containers. These are thick, rich and moisturizing. They have a heavy texture and, because of the heavy coverage, make it unnecessary to use a concealer. Thick cream-based foundations are often used for theatre and television makeup or photographic portraits. Some makeup artists may use a cream-based foundation for special occasions, however the disadvantage is that it can cause blockage of the pores due to the thick consistency.

Powder Face powder comes in compact cases in a cake form with a puff, or loosely, also with a puff. Compact powders are useful for touching up makeup. Loose powder is best applied with the makeup.

Powder foundation (See mineral makeup below)

Eye shadows These come in a container either singly or as a duo or trio of colours in palettes. Eye shadow can be purchased in a case with a combination of colour eye shadow palettes together with blusher and lipstick.

Eyebrow pencils and eye liners These come as pencils and liquid liners. Pencils are best used for older women, while eye liners are more suitable for younger people.

Eyebrow pencil sharpeners These are designed for eyebrow and eye liner pencils. Ordinary pencil sharpeners will ruin an eyebrow pencil.

Blushers These come in cream or powder form. Rouge is a cream-based blusher and was popular from the decades of the 1920s through to the 1960s. Some older women still like to use a rouge-based blusher and these should be applied before powder. During the Second World War, lipstick was substituted for rouge, due to the shortage of cosmetics. This was a good idea at the time, as it matched the colour of the lipstick worn on the lips. Some older women of that generation still use this method. Powder-based blushers are more popular and more suitable for women of all ages.

Lip liners These come in soft pencils or in liquid pens. The pencil liners are easy to apply and they feel soft, like a lipstick, when applied.

Lipstick and lip gloss These come mainly in tubes but also in palettes and small containers. Lipstick should be applied to the lips with a lip brush. Lip gloss can be applied over the lipstick colour for a more glossy depth, or it can be worn on its own.

Lip liner pencil applied to the lips and blended with a lip gloss makes a good combination for women who do not like to wear a lot of lip colour.

Mineral makeup A new trend in cosmetics exploding onto the beauty market at present is that of mineral cosmetics. These products are packaged as powder foundations, blushers, eye shadows and lipsticks. They have become popular because the minerals contained in them claim to have a soothing effect on the skin for some consumers as they claim not to contain the harsh chemicals, dyes, fragrances and preservatives of traditional cosmetics. They claim to have the ability to leave the skin with a natural glow, not to clog the pores in the skin and in some cases they claim to sooth minor inflammation for some sufferers. Not all mineral cosmetics are what they claim to be as some may contain synthetics (e.g. parabean preservatives). The 'true' mineral products do not have these preservatives. Read the labels before purchase and be careful not to get drawn in by the advertising and the slick 'attractive' marketing.

The most popular product in mineral cosmetics is a powdered foundation. It comes as a loose powder and caters for all skin types. The powder is applied similarly to ordinary face powder with a brush. This product can be used as an alternative to using powder and foundation separately.

As the mineral cosmetics have been on the market only a short time, I have not been able to complete clinical trials before publication of this book. The 'true' mineral powder may be an alternative for frail older women and for those with sensitive skin.

Remember, no matter how enticing advertised products may be, some people can still have a sensitivity or allergic reaction.

Step by step in makeup application
Light touch
(Suitable for older women, those with sensitive skins, and those who do not like wearing a lot of colour makeup)

1 Apply a tinted moisture cream
2 Apply powder (optional)
3 Apply neutral eye shadow if desired
4 Apply lipstick

Light day makeup (1)

1   Apply a tinted moisture cream
2   Apply powder
3   Apply two eye shadow colours
4   Add a touch of blusher
5   Apply lipstick

Light day makeup (2)

1   Apply foundation
2   Apply powder
3   Apply two eye shadow colours
4   Apply blusher
5   Apply lipstick

Day makeup, full application

1   Apply foundation
2   Apply concealer
3   Apply powder
4   Apply two to three eye shadows
5   Apply eye liner if desired
6   Apply eyebrow pencil or shadow colour
7   Apply mascara
8   Apply blusher
9   Apply lip liner and lipstick

For evening wear (from teens to mid 30s)

Younger people in this age group can use shimmery eye shadows giving a touch of glitter around the eyes. Eye liners can be worn a little darker or lighter and lips can be painted with glossy sensual colours. Cream-based blushers can add extra gloss to a younger complexion. Coloured mascara or extra mascara can be worn to accentuate the eyelashes and eyes.

Makeup application tips for older women

Applying makeup to the skin of an older person is very much the same as it is for a younger person, except that the skin is looser and lines and furrows have begun to appear. For some women, when applying a foundation, eye shadow and eyebrow colours, the skin may need to be stretched and held firm. By doing this, the colour on the eyelids, eyebrow line, cheek area and the lips will not look too dark or thick when makeup is applied over these furrows and lines. By holding the skin firm with one hand, using the other hand to apply the makeup, the colour is easy to apply smoothly, giving the woman a natural overall look. For some older women, it is best to follow the day steps for most makeup applications. Some older women would prefer the light touch or one of the two light day makeup routines as mentioned above rather than the full day application. For evening wear, apply makeup as for day wear and add a little more depth of colour to the eyes and lips. If using an eye shadow colour, brush a little extra colour around the eyelid line and a little at the corners of the eye. Add a little more depth of colour to the eyebrows. A darker shade of lipstick with a touch of gloss may suit some older women for evening wear.

Conclusion

In conclusion, I trust that I have achieved what I set out to do in writing this book. My aim was to share my experience with you and instil a sense of confidence for the carer working with the aged and infirm and for those using cosmetic treatments at home. I hope that I have achieved my aim and that you will find the information useful.

Useful websites

The websites listed below are current at the time of my research on 30 June 2008 before publication.

Apply Makeup. Com (June 2008) Asian makeup
www.applymakeup.com

Eyebrow Biz (June 2008) Eyebrow and Makeup Tips
www.eyebrowz.com

Ayurvedic Cure (2008) Makeup for dark skin
www.ayurvediccure.com/makeup_darkskin.htm

Mineral makeup
www.webmd.com/skin-beauty/features/the-lowdown-on-mineral
-makeup

Wedding Makeup
www.usabride.com/wedplan/a_makeup_tips.html

Glossary

Abrasive treatment	Where a coarse substance or applicator is used to rub, scrape or wear away dead skin cells on the surface of the body.
Accentuate	To emphasize, make prominent, to stand out, be noticed.
Blemish	Flaw, defect, stain.
Classic (colours)	Prominent colours used in fashion which do not become out-dated. E.g. white, black, navy, grey, taupe, red.
Colour coding	To screen certain colours, including 'classic' and 'signature' colours that

complement the overall colour tone of an individual. This includes makeup, dress sense and hair style.

Elements   Created by nature: air, water, earth, fire. Atmospheric agents: storm, wind, rain, pollutants. Home and office buildings: electrical heating and cooling systems.

Features   Includes the eyes, eyebrows, nose, cheeks, lips, chin and face 'overall' profile.

Formula   A list of cosmetics suitable for the right skin, hair and eye colour and a sequence for use.

Highlight   To bring out, show off and accentuate a certain feature.

Lip line   Outer edges of the lips.

Makeover   Full makeup application. Can include a new hair style and wardrobe.

Makeup   Combination of coloured cosmetics used to colour features on the face for improvement, theatre work and photography.

Matt   Having no shine or gloss.

Neutral   Containing no colour.

Origin   Ancestry, parentage, starting point.

Palette   1 Thin board or slab for mixing colours.

2 Small palette-like containers that contain colours of eye shadow, blushers, lipsticks either singular, duo, trio or in one large palette container.

Pastel   Light shade of colour.

Pollution   Contamination of the environment.

Recede	To distance, to hide away.
Rejuvenate	To freshen, to smooth, make young again.
Seep	Ooze out.
Shade	To give shadow or darken a feature or blemish.
Signature (colours)	Certain colours which suit an individual and accentuate their best assets and features. E.g. pink, blue, yellow, green, etc.
Skin tone	'Colour shades' of the skin.
Spatula	Flat applicator used to apply cosmetics.
Technique	Mechanical skill as in 'art' or presentation.
Tone	Tint or shade of colour.

Bibliography

Bean, A., Broadman, S., Crawley, H., *et al.* (1997) *Eating for Good Health.* Sydney: Readers Digest. (Original work published 1995).

Burke, K. (1996) *Great Skin for Life.* London: Hamlyn.

Campsie, J. (1997) *Marie Claire.* Sydney: Murdoch Books.

Chevalier, A. (2001) *Encyclopaedia of Medicinal Plants.* London: Dorling Kindersley.

Frankle, R.T. and Owen, A. (1986) *Nutrition in the Community,* 3rd edition. St Louis: Mosby. (Original work published 1978).

Gawkrodger, D.J. (2002) *Dermatology,* 3rd edition. Edinburgh: Churchill-Livingstone.

Hale, T. (1996) *The Hale Clinic Guide to Good Health.* London: Kyle Cathie.

Miller, B.F. and Keane, C.B. (1983) *Saunders Encyclopaedia and Dictionary of Medicine, Nursing, and Allied Health.* Philadelphia: WB Saunders.

Ostrov, R. (1999) *Solving Skin Problems.* London: Marshall.

Polunin, M. (1997) *Healing Foods.* London: Dorling Kindersley.

Robinson, J. and Barrett, K. (1999) *Caring for your Feet.* Sydney: Choice Books.

Short, K. (1991) *Vitamin and Mineral Decoder.* Melbourne: Dynamo House.

Stanway, P. (2000) *The Feel-Good Facelift, The Natural Way to Look Good and Feel Younger.* London: Kyle Cathie.

Wildwood, C. (1998) *The Encyclopaedia of Healing Plants.* London: Piatkus.

Winter, R. (2005) *A Consumer's Dictionary of Cosmetic Ingredients.* New York: Three Rivers Press. (Original work published 1978).

Worwood, V.A. (1990) *The Fragrant Pharmacy.* London: Macmillan.